Recent Results in Cancer Research

Fortschritte der Krebsforschung

Progrès dans les recherches sur le cancer

5

Edited by

Springer-Verlag · New York, Inc. 1966

Recent Results in Cancer Research

Fortschritte der Krebsforschung

Progrès dans les recherches sur le cancer

5

Edited by

V. G. Allfrey, New York · M. Allgöwer, Chur · K. H. Bauer, Heidelberg · I. Berenblum, Rehovoth · F. Bergel, London · J. Bernard, Paris · W. Bernhard, Villejuif · N. N. Blokhin, Moskva · H. E. Bock, Tübingen · P. Bucalossi, Milano · A. V. Chaklin, Moskva · M. Chorazy, Gliwice · G. J. Cunningham, London · W. Dameshek, Boston · M. Dargent, Lyon · G. Della Porta, Milano · P. Denoix, Villejuif · R. Dulbecco, San Diego · H. Eagle, New York · R. Eker, Oslo · P. Grabar, Paris · H. Hamperl, Bonn · R. J. C. Harris, London · E. Hecker, Heidelberg · R. Herbeuval, Nancy · J. Higginson, Lyon · W. C. Hueper, Bethesda · H. Isliker, Lausanne · D. A. Karnofsky, New York · J. Kieler, København · G. Klein, Stockholm · H. Koprowski, Philadelphia · L. G. Koss, New York · G. Martz, Zürich · G. Mathé, Paris · O. Mühlbock, Amsterdam · G. T. Pack, New York · V. R. Potter, Madison · A. B. Sabin, Cincinnati · L. Sachs, Rehovoth · E. A. Saxén, Helsinki · W. Szybalski, Madison · H. Tagnon, Bruxelles · R. M. Taylor, Toronto · A. Tissières, Genève · E. Uehlinger, Zürich · R. W. Wissler, Chicago · T. Yoshida, Tokyo · L. A. Zilber, Moskva

Editor in chief

P. Rentchnick, Genève

Springer-Verlag New York Inc. 1966

The Thymus

Its Role in Immune Responses, Leukaemia Development and Carcinogenesis

Donald Metcalf

With a Foreword by Sir Macfarlane Burnet

With 44 Figures

Springer-Verlag · New York, Inc. 1966

Dr. Donald Metcalf, M. D., Assistant Director, Head — Cancer Research Unit. Walter and Eliza Hall Institute of Medical Research, University of Melbourne, Victoria / Australia.

Sir Macfarlane Burnet, M. D., Ph. D., F. R. S., Emeritus Professor, University of Melbourne. Formerly Director of Walter and Eliza Hall Institute of Medical Research, University of Melbourne, Victoria/Australia.

Sponsored by the Swiss League against Cancer

ISBN-13: 978-3-642-46046-3 e-ISBN-13: 978-3-642-46044-9
DOI: 10.1007/978-3-642-46044-9

Softcover reprint of the hardcover 1st edition 1966

Library of Congress Catalog Card Number 65-6383.

 Title No. 7469

To Josephine

Foreword

The sudden burst of interest in the thymus during the last five years more than justifies the appearance of a monograph on those aspects of its function which bear particularly on immunity and the processes associated with the development of malignant disease. Of those who are actively working in the field I believe that Dr. DONALD METCALF is uniquely suited to produce such a work. His demonstration of a lymphocytosis stimulating factor from thymic tissue in 1956 was almost the first evidence of physiological activity by the thymus. He has played an important part in the analysis of the leukaemogenic process in mice and his recent work on thymic grafting has been almost disconcertingly productive of new ideas.

I feel confident that this monograph will be of great value to a wide range of investigators and teachers interested in obtaining a clear summary of the present position. Incidentally, Dr. METCALF has provided a well chosen sample of factual material from which others who may wish to question some of his speculations, can draw their own conclusions. He has been careful to keep the observational and experimental facts clearly distinct from theoretical matters but has not shirked from making his contribution to the current ferment of immunological theory. Personally I am sorry that he is not more sympathetic to my own view which would endow the thymus with the censorship function of eliminating unsuitable immunocytes and provide a rationale for that „slaughter of the innocents“ amongst thymic lymphocytes which has been one of the most striking of METCALF's discoveries.

Perhaps one of the most important virtues of the monograph is its recognition that there is still much to be learnt about the thymus. It is one of the delights of biological research that one never reaches final conclusions. Almost certainly there are endocrine aspects of thymic function yet to be discovered and I suspect that its relevance to autoimmune disease is greater than has yet been established. Whatever may develop in the future I feel that this monograph provides a splendid picture of the foundation on which all future studies must be based.

Melbourne University, December, 1965. F. M. BURNET

Preface

The thymus has had a chequered past and it was not until the mid 1940's that the work of FURTH followed by that of LAW and KAPLAN, established the first solid fact about the thymus — that thymectomy prevents the development of lymphoid leukaemia in mice. When the author commenced working on the thymus in the mid 1950's as a result of chance observations on the lymphocytosis stimulating activity of various types of leukaemic sera, it was still possible to list significant papers on the function of the thymus (with the exception of the mouse leukaemia work) on the fingers of one hand. In 1961 a dramatic change occurred in the fortunes of the thymus with the independent demonstration by MILLER and by GOOD and his colleagues of the immunological effects of neonatal thymectomy. Since this time, there has been an exponential growth of work on the thymus, until at the present time (1965) it is becoming difficult to keep abreast of the growing literature.

This monograph has been written as a somewhat oversimplified account of the present status of knowledge of the thymus in the hope that it will prove of some value as an introduction to the thymus for colleagues in allied fields and for younger colleagues who are about to enter what is becoming an extremely complex field. This work is not intended to be an exhaustive review of the literature on the thymus, and the author apologises in advance to those of his colleagues whose excellent contributions have not been discussed in the following pages.

At times the author has reached beyond established fact in an attempt to fit just a few more pieces in the puzzle. It is hoped that such speculations will be met with the response intended — scepticism and further experiments.

DONALD METCALF

Table of Contents

Chapter 1

The Structure of the Thymus

The thymus is a large lymphoid organ located in most species in the upper anterior mediastinum of the chest. In some species like the guinea pig and fowl it occupies a subcutaneous site in the cervical region and in Australian marsupials two thymus glands are present—one cervical and one thoracic. To be more exact, the thymus is not a bi-lobed organ but rather a pair of organs which, when in the thoracic region, become firmly bound together in the mid-line. In the cervical region the dual nature of the thymus glands is more apparent for the glands are arranged in a chain of lobules on either side of the neck. Thus various species possess either two or four thymus glands but in the interests of simplicity these organs hereafter will be referred to simply as "the thymus".

Embryologically the epithelial elements of the thymus are believed to arise from outgrowths of the third and fourth branchial pouches, around which mesodermal elements aggregate. It is likely that these mesodermal elements give rise to the thymus capsule, the thymus inter-lobular septae and possibly the reticulum cells of the thymus. Some doubt remains as to the origin of the lymphoid cells of the thymus. The *in vitro* experiments of AUERBACH (1961) strongly suggest that during embryological development the epithelial cells of the thymus, under the inductive influence of the surrounding mesenchymal cells, divide to form the precursors of the lymphoid cells. If this is so, then the situation must change after birth for it has been shown clearly (see below) that in post natal life most of the lymphoid cells of the thymus are continually replaced by new blood-borne cells, which are probably of bone marrow origin.

The typical thymus in most mammals is a large whitish grey, apparently bi-lobed, organ with a curiously avascular appearance. Thymic blood vessels are small in size and most appear to arise from the internal mammary arteries. There is some doubt whether or not a true lymphatic drainage system is present in the thymus but a limited degree of drainage may occur to the parathymic lymph nodes.

The absolute size of the thymus varies widely from one species to another and in most species the thymus is broken up by fibrous septae into lobules, each lobule containing a central area, the medulla, and a surrounding cortex of lymphoid cells. It is a striking feature of the thymus that although the size of the whole organ varies widely in different species, the absolute size of the thymic lobule is remarkably similar in all species. This uniformity in lobular size is particularly evident with respect to the width of the lymphoid cortex in the thymic lobules (Fig. 1) and suggests that there may be a critical size limit for the width of the cortex in relation to the size of the medulla.

The mouse thymus has been studied in more detail than the thymus in other species and the general characteristics of the growth of this organ will now be

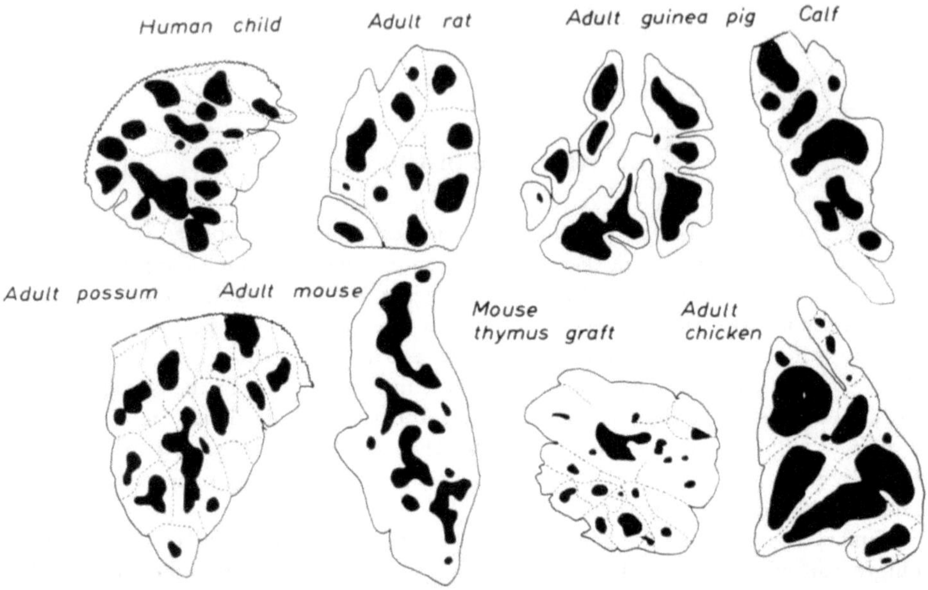

Fig. 1. Camera lucida drawings at same magnification of sections of the thymus from various species. Note the similar architectural pattern and size of the thymic lobules in different species. Black areas represent medullary tissue

described. However with minor variations, the following description of age changes in the thymus applies equally to the thymus in all species.

The thymus becomes lymphoid late in foetal life, and the organ rapidly increases in size after birth, reaching a maximum weight between the fourth and sixth weeks of age (adolescence). After this time a characteristic loss of weight occurs (age involution) which proceeds rapidly for the first few months, then continues at a very much slower rate for the remainder of the life of the animal (METCALF, 1960 a). At most ages the ratio of cortical tissue area to medullary tissue area in the thymus is constant (9 : 1), but in old age thymus atrophy tends to affect the lymphoid cortex more severely than the medulla. Thus in humans in old age, little may be found of the thymus other than islands of epithelial cells in a mass of fatty tissue which has infiltrated the original space occupied by the lymphoid cortex in earlier life (HAMMAR, 1921).

Much has been written on the apparent disappearance of the thymus in adult humans. To a large degree these descriptions are in error for the human thymus remains a distinct and sizeable organ throughout middle age. Most earlier data on humans were derived from studies on autopsy material or on the thymus at operation. It is now appreciated that rapid atrophy of the thymus occurs within 24 hours of the onset of any serious illness and that the usual appearance of the thymus at post mortem or at operation is not a true indication of the size of the thymus in normal persons of the same age (BOYD, 1932). The true size of the human thymus can only be determined by a study of the organ in cases of sudden or accidental death, in previously healthy persons.

The age involution weight loss in the thymus after adolescence is unique for this organ and no parallel weight loss changes occur at this time in any other lymphoid or haemopoietic organ in the body (Fig. 2) (METCALF, 1964). In mice it can be shown

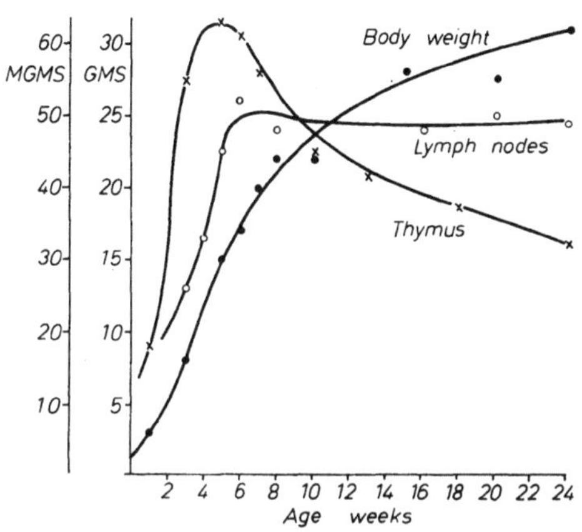

Fig. 2

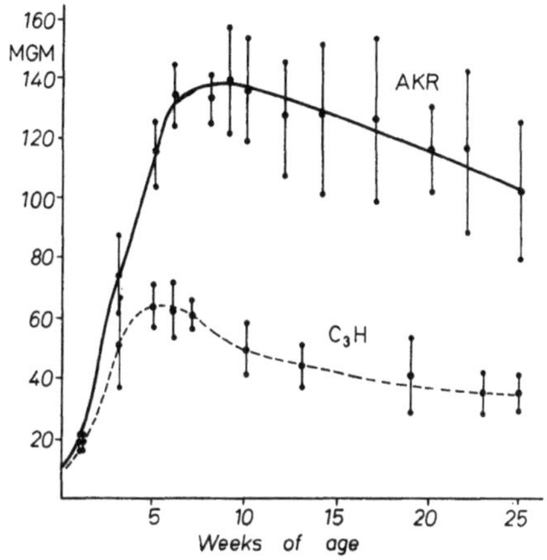

Fig. 3

Fig. 2. Changes with age in C3H mice of body weight (in Gm) and the weights of the thymus and subcutaneous lymph nodes (in mgm)

Fig. 3. Age related changes in the weight of the thymus in female AKR and C3H mice

that the female thymus is heavier than the male at all ages and that in different species of inbred mice with the same body weight, the thymus exhibits characteristic strain differences in weight (Fig. 3), (METCALF, 1960 a). Both these features of the thymus again are not paralleled by comparable sex or strain differences in the weights of other lymphoid organs.

There is a fundamental difference between the thymus and other lymphoid organs in the response of these organs to antigenic stimulation. This is seen clearly in animals raised under germfree (that is relatively antigen-free) conditions. In such animals, the thymus is normal in size but the lymph nodes and spleen lymphoid follicles are quite atrophic (THORBECKE et al., 1957; GORDON, 1959). Conversely, antigenic stimulation has been shown to increase lymph node and spleen weights and cellular activity but has no effect on the thymus size or cellular activity (METCALF, 1964). In severe natural or experimental infections, the thymus commonly atrophies at the same time as the nonthymic lymphoid organs hypertrophy. These studies have made it clear that antigenic stimulation is the primary proliferative stimulus for nonthymic lymphoid tissues but the size and cellular activity of the thymus appear to be independent of antigenic stimulation. Probably related to this lack of dependence of thymus growth or function on antigenic stimulation are the absence of lymphoid follicles and germinal centres from the normal thymus and the fact that plasma cells are rare (less than 0.1% of total lymphoid cells) in the thymic parenchyma. In certain disease states, for example myasthenia gravis in humans, and auto immune haemolytic anaemia in mice, lymphoid follicles and germinal centres do occur in the thymus but in such conditions these follicles are always located in the medullary region, not in the lymphoid cortex.

At first sight the histological structure of the thymus (Fig. 4) appears deceptively simple but more detailed study has revealed it to be highly complex. The thymic

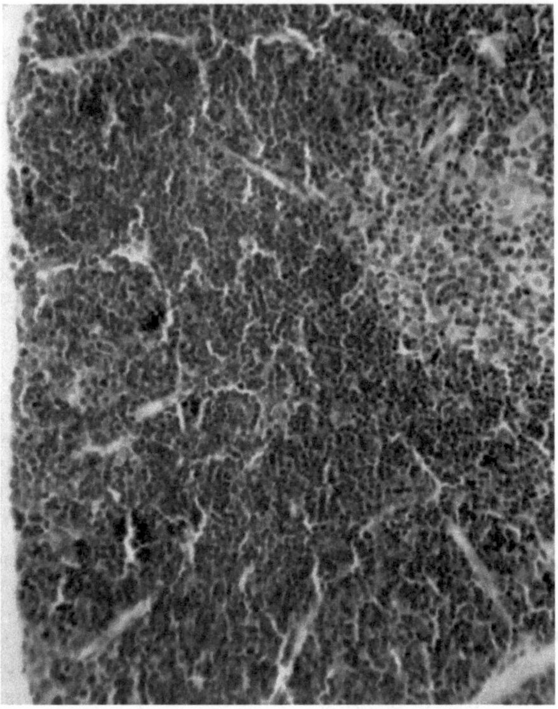

Fig. 4. Photomicrograph of portion of the normal C3H mouse thymus. Note cortical region of densely packed lymphoid cells and the lighter staining medullary tissue containing epithelial cells. H and E ×200

lobule is best visualised as being basically a sponge of epithelial and reticulum cells, in the interstices of which are embedded aggregates of tightly packed lymphoid cells. The epithelial spongework is densest in the central region of the lobule—giving this area (the medulla) an almost non lymphoid appearance. In fact, the medulla is composed of epithelial cells, mixed with various types of reticulum cells and some lymphoid cells. The morphological appearance of the epithelial cell aggregates in the medulla varies from one species to another. In some, such as the human, they are aggregated in whorled patterns (the (Hassall's corpuscles) but in others, such as the mouse, the epithelial cells may lie singly or in clumps of polygonal cells or may occasionally be columnar in shape with a ciliated border and be arranged in small vesicles (Arnesen, 1958). The significance of these different morphological forms is not understood but they may be related to different functional states of the cells or possibly indicate a distinct heterogeneity in this cell population. The epithelial cells are united by desmosome bridges, are not phagocytic and appear to secrete a PAS-positive material which may be seen in the cytoplasm as fine granules or dense blobs (CLARK, 1963; HOSHINO, 1963).

Recently CLARK (1965) has made a more detailed electron microscopic study of the epithelial cells of the mouse thymus. He observed a developmental sequence with increasing age in the secretory products of medullary epithelial cells. Before birth these cells contain basophilic granules in the Golgi region of the cell but after birth clusters of vacuoles develop, some containing basophilic granules. With increasing age of the animal large coalescent vacuoles develop and contain secretory material which gives a PAS-positive staining reaction, and may be sulphated mucopolysaccharide or glycoprotein. CLARK also observed that such cells concentrated S_{35}-sulphate and C_{14}-glucosamine from one to four hours after administration and in autoradiographs, the label was observed over the vacuoles in the cytoplasm.

In the cortex the epithelial cells are elongated flattened cells which radiate out from the medulla along the radial vessels and enclose the outer aspects of the lobule. In effect these epithelial cells form the frame work of a relatively cell-tight sponge enclosing spaces of variable size (Fig. 5). This cell sponge system is not complete and

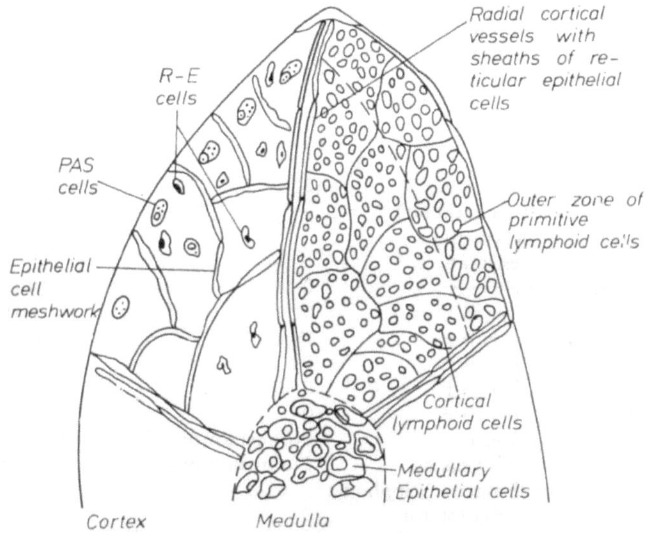

Fig. 5. Schematic diagram of portion of the thymus showing medullary epithelial cells and the spongework of ret'-ular epithelial cells in the cortex. Interstices of cortical spongework are packed with lymphoid and reticulo-endothelial cells

gaps are present in the tubular arrangement of epithelial cells along the radial vessels, particularly in the outer sub-capsular regions of the cortex (CLARK, 1963; HOSHINO, 1963; WEISS, 1963). It is not certain whether or not the flattened reticular epithelial cells of this cortical meshwork are functionally identical with the epithelial cells of the medulla but they at least give the same types of histochemical reactions (Table 1) (METCALF, 1964). However CLARK (1965) has produced evidence suggesting that the cortical epithelial cells may differ from those in the medulla. In the electron microscope, the secretory vacuoles of cortical epithelial cells have a characteristically different appearance from those in medullary epithelial cells and the cortical epithelial cells do not concentrate S_{35}-sulphate or C_{14}-glucosamine as do the epithelial cells of the medulla.

Table 1. *Comparison of Cytological Features of Various Thymic Cell Types in C57Bl Mice*

	PAS phagocytic reticulum cells	Reticular epithelial cells of perivascular sheath	Medullary epithelial cells
Location	Cortex outer third	Cortex	Medulla
Shape	Rounded	Flattened, stellate	Variable
Nucleus	Single, round or oval. Mean diameter 5.8 μ.	Single, elongated oval. Mean diameter 4.7 μ.	Single, round or oval. Mean diameter 7.6 μ.
Cytoplasm	Bulky. Increases with age. Yellow pigment	Attenuated. No change with age. No pigment	Variable. No change with age. No pigment
PAS Reaction	Intense. Granular diastase & RDE resistant	Occasional granules or aggregates	Variable. Small granules to large aggregates. Diastase & RDE resistant
Histochemistry of cytoplasm			
Eosin	0	+	+ to +++
Pyronine	++++ (nongranular) RNA-ase resistant	0	0 to +++ RNA-ase resistant
Alkaline phosphatase	++++	0	0 (some +++)
Acid phosphatase	++++	0	0 (few ++)
Esterase	++++	++	0 to ++++
5-Nucleotidase	++++	0	0
A.T.P.-ase	++++	0	0 to ++
6-Glucosephosphatase	++++	0	0 (some ++)
Toluidine blue	Green	No metachromasia	No metachromasia
Wrights stain	Faint metachromatic stippling	No metachromasia	No metachromasia
Feulgen	0 Except for phagocytosed nuclear debris	0	0
Mitotic activity	Rare in adult.	Not seen.	Uncommon in adult.
Lymphocyte phagocytosis	30% of cells in normal thymus	Not phagocytic	Not phagocytic
Mitotic activity in adjacent lymphocytes	Yes	No	No

The cortical epithelial spongework is filled by dense aggregates of lymphoid cells. These thymic lymphoid cells appear slightly smaller than the lymph node lymphocytes and it has been suggested that this may be the result of tighter cell packing in

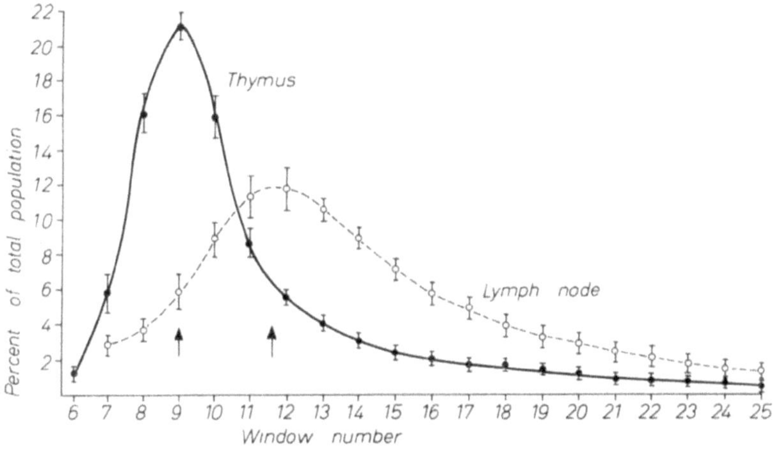

Fig. 6. Coulter counter analysis of two months old normal C57Bl mouse thymus and subcutaneous lymph node cell suspensions. Large peaks in both curves represent small lymphocytes, which are larger and more heterogeneous in the lymph node than in the thymus. Each point mean value from six mice, vertical bars the standard deviations of values

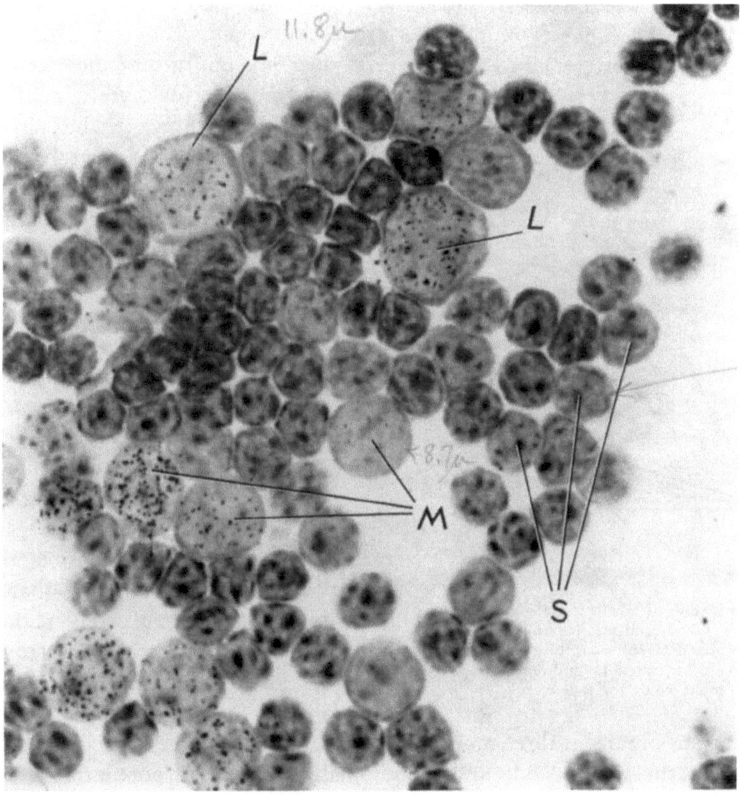

Fig. 7. Smear of normal AKR mouse thymic lymphocytes, showing large (L), medium (M) and small (S) lymphocytes. Autoradiograph made one hour after labelling with tritiated thymidine. Note that only the large and medium cells have taken up isotope. Exposure time 31 days. Giemsa stain ×1400 (reduced to $^{9}/_{10}$)

the thymus than in the lymph node. However we have recently made size measurements on the cell volumes of mouse thymic and lymph node small lymphocytes using an electronic Coulter counter. It is quite clear from the results (Fig. 6) that thymic small lymphocytes really are smaller than lymph node small lymphocytes. Moreover there appears to be a greater degree of heterogeneity in the size of lymph node small lymphocytes than in thymic small lymphocytes.

The cortical lymphoid cells make up 90% of the weight of the organ and cytological studies on the mouse thymus have revealed that three types of lymphocyte are present in the lymphoid aggregates—large, medium and small (Fig. 7). In thymus cell smears from AKR mice the frequency of these cell types is—1% large (greater than 11 μ, total cell diameter) 10% medium (7—11 μ) and 89% small (less than 7 μ). These three cell types form a cell sequence with the large cells dividing to form medium cells which in turn divide to form small lymphocytes.

The thymic cortical lymphoid cells exhibit intense mitotic activity but mitoses are uncommon in the medullary lymphoid cells. Recent autoradiographic studies using tritiated thymidine labelling have indicated that in the two months old AKR thymus, the large lymphocytes divide every 6.8 hours and the medium lymphocytes every 8.2 hours (METCALF and WIADROWSKI, 1966). Most thymic small lymphocytes appear to be non-dividing cells, and only 2% of these cells directly incorporate tritiated thymidine. The term "non-dividing cell" does not imply that these cells are incapable of mitosis, for thymic small lymphocytes have been shown to be activated *in vitro* by the addition of phytohaemagglutinin (MARSHALL, personal communication). It appears, however, that few thymic small lymphocytes normally exhibit their inherent capacity to proliferate—at least during their stay in the thymus. Thymic small lymphocytes appear to be produced by the asymmetrical division of medium lymphocytes and the replacement rate of thymic small lymphocytes is extremely rapid—the vast majority of the population of small lymphocytes in the mouse thymus being replaced every three to four days. The replacement rate of the thymic population of small lymphocytes is far more rapid than that of small lymphocyte populations in the lymph nodes, spleen, blood or bone marrow. Fig. 8 indicates the accumulation of tritiated thymidine labelled (newly formed) small lymphocytes in various organs in three months old C57Bl mice and these data suggest a turnover time for the lymph node and blood small lymphocyte population of possibly 30 to 100 days with the bone marrow small lymphocyte population replacement time lying somewhere between this and the 3—4 days for cells in the thymus (METCALF, 1965). Data from tritiated thymidine studies in the rat confirm the relatively slow

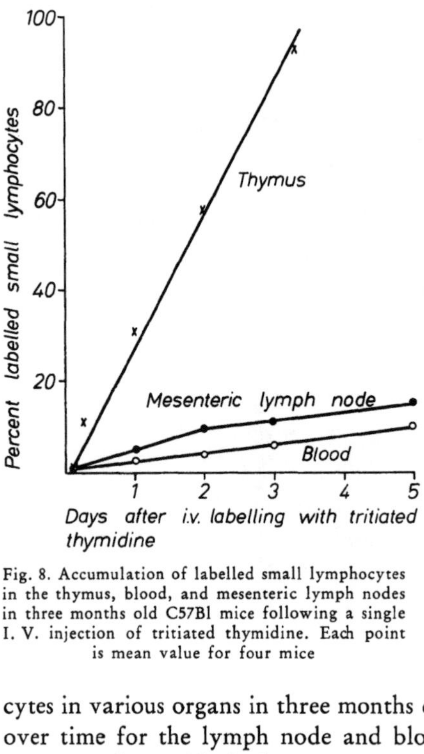

Fig. 8. Accumulation of labelled small lymphocytes in the thymus, blood, and mesenteric lymph nodes in three months old C57Bl mice following a single I. V. injection of tritiated thymidine. Each point is mean value for four mice

replacement time of the population of small lymphocytes in the body, compared with that in the thymus (LITTLE *et al.*, 1962).

The mitotic activity of thymic lymphoid cells may also be measured by direct mitotic counts on thymus sections or thymus cell smears. The results obtained by both methods suggest that mitotic indices are 5—10 times higher in thymic lymphoid cells than in lymph node or spleen lymphocytes (KINDRED, 1938; ANDREASEN and CHRISTENSEN, 1949; METCALF and NAKAMURA, 1962). Data from human tissues suggest a similar difference in proliferative activity (METCALF, 1964).

However the data from mitotic indices and from small lymphocyte replacement times are deceptive in suggesting that thymic cells divide much more rapidly than lymphocytes elsewhere in the body. In the mouse and rat, tritiated thymidine labelling data from antigenically stimulated spleen lymphoid follicles indicate that the primitive lymphoid cells in this location divide every 5—7 hours—that is at about the same rate as thymic lymphoid cells (FLIEDNER et al., 1964; HANNA, 1964).

The true situation appears to be that lymphocyte proliferative activity in an organ like the lymph node is very variable, and depends on the current level of antigenic stimulation. In the germfree state, lymph nodes exhibit minimal proliferative activity but under conditions of maximum antigen stimulation the primitive lymphoid cells are able to proliferate as rapidly as the corresponding cells in the thymus. The so-called "normal" animal occupies an intermediate position, being normally subject to a continuous low level of antigenic stimulation. In the normal thymus, the primitive lymphoid cells (particularly the medium lymphocytes) do proliferate more rapidly than corresponding cells in the lymph nodes or the spleen, but the difference in proliferative rates is probably only a two to threefold one. The probable reasons why direct mitotic counts on lymph node populations give much lower mitotic indices than for thymic cells are 1. that the percentage of primitive cells is lower in the lymph node than in the thymus (e.g. in C57Bl mice 0.5% large and 2.6% medium lymphocytes in the subcutaneous lymph node versus 1% and 10% medium lymphocytes in the thymus)—this difference being the result of the different life spans of the small lymphocytes in the two tissues; 2. that many so-called primitive "lymphoid" cells in lymph nodes are in fact not giving rise to lymphocytes but to other cell types, primarily plasma cells, and 3. that some primitive cells in lymph nodes may die before or during mitosis, for it is well known that pyknotic cells are common in germinal centres, and labelled lymphocyte nuclear material (presumably from primitive lymphoid cells) rapidly appears in the phagocytic cells of germinal centres (FLIEDNER et al., 1964).

The relative rates of division of lymphoid cells in the thymus and other organs have been discussed at some length because of some confusion in the past over this question and because the rate of proliferation of thymic lymphoid cells may have a bearing, as will be seen later, on the peculiar susceptibility of thymic lymphoid cells to the development of neoplasia.

The mitotic activity of thymic lymphoid cells is not constant throughout life. In the mouse mitotic indices of the primitive lymphoid cells are highest in the neonatal period and fall during the first few weeks of life (Fig. 9). There is a further pronounced fall occurring at the commencement of age involution but thereafter mitotic indices remain at a relatively constant level throughout adult life (NAKAMURA and METCALF, 1961). The fall in thymic mitotic activity at the time of age involution is probably responsible in part for the fall in weight of the organ at this time, although a reduction in the volume of the epithelial and reticulum cell sponge may also be involved. Where age involution is delayed, as in the female AKR mouse thymus, there is also a delay in the fall of primitive cell mitotic activity.

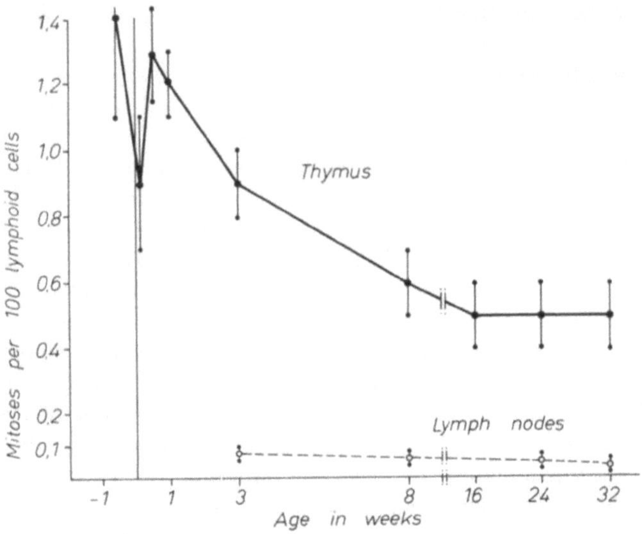

Fig. 9. Frequency of mitoses in cell smears from the thymus and subcutaneous lymph nodes of C3H mice at various ages. Each point is mean value of eight mice; vertical bars are standard deviations for each group

In the mouse, female thymic mitotic indices are slightly higher than in the male, and mitotic indices are higher in some mouse strains than in others (Nakamura and Metcalf, 1961). For example, thymic mitotic indices in high leukaemia strain AKR mice are consistently higher than in low leukaemia strain C3H mice at all ages.

In the human thymus there appears to be less age fluctuation in mitotic activity, and at least throughout childhood (1—15 years) mitotic indices are relatively constant (Metcalf, 1964). Little data are at present available for the adult human thymus but in a few samples examined in this laboratory, thymic mitotic indices seemed similar to those in childhood. This suggests that in humans although the thymus may become smaller with advancing age, those thymic lymphoid cells which remain may continue to proliferate at a rapid rate.

In the assessment of lymphocyte mitotic activity the measurement of mitotic indices appears to be a more sensitive technique than determination of cell proliferation rates from tritiated thymidine autoradiography. For example autoradiographic data cannot discriminate between the mitotic activity of two months old male and female AKR thymic lymphoid cells yet mitotic indices determinations show a clear sex difference in mitotic activity at this age.

Potentially, tritiated thymidine studies should be of greatest value in determining the proliferative patterns of the primitive thymic lymphoid cells—for example in determining what proportion of cells divide to give rise to parental type or daughter type offspring. When a single pulse intravenous label of tritiated thymidine is given, only those primitive cells in DNA synthesis (the S phase of the mitotic cycle) at the time of labelling will incorporate tritiated thymidine which is a specific precursor of DNA. It should then be possible to follow the appearance of label in the subsequent offspring of these cells and thereby to analyse in detail the sequence of cell divisions in the thymus. Unfortunately such studies are rendered impossible by the phenomenon of reutilization of label (MITCHELL, McDONALD and NOSSAL, 1963; METCALF and WIADROWSKI, 1966). Some cells which initially take up label, break down and release isotope which is incorporated into other previously unlabelled cells. Hence it becomes impossible to determine whether any given labelled cell is the daughter of a labelled cell or has merely acquired label by reutilization. Tritiated thymidine studies do allow certain generalisations to be made. In the mouse, large lymphocytes divide to form both large lymphocyte and medium lymphocyte offspring. In turn medium lymphocytes divide to form both medium lymphocyte and small lymphocyte offspring. The large majority of small lymphocytes are non-dividing cells but the population of small lymphocytes in the thymus rapidly becomes labelled because of the generation of new small lymphocytes from labelled medium lymphocytes.

LEBLOND and SAINTE MARIE (1960) have made a mathematical analysis of thymic lymphoid cells in the rat and have proposed an elaborate sequence of cell divisions to account for the observed proportions of large, medium and small lymphocytes in the thymus. This system envisages a number of subclasses of cells within each of the three cell categories. Tritiated thymidine data are not incompatible with this system but are not precise enough to provide a positive confirmation of the existence of these subclasses.

In general terms, it can be said that the large and medium cells are self sustaining by virtue of asymmetrical divisions. Thus alternate large lymphocyte divisions give rise to either two large lymphocyte offspring or two medium lymphocyte offspring, and alternate medium lymphocyte divisions give rise to either two medium lymphocyte offspring or to two small lymphocyte offspring. Since the relative proportions of large to medium to small lymphocytes remain constant, this asymmetrical division of large and medium lymphocytes cannot produce exactly 50% parental type and 50% daughter type offspring or the population size of medium lymphocytes would increase progressively. A slight excess of medium lymphocyte offspring must be small lymphocytes or else some medium lymphocytes must die at, or soon after, mitosis. Whatever the exact process, a slow deficit of medium lymphocytes develops (at approximately the rate of 1 in 8 medium lymphocyte divisions in the AKR thymus) which is made good by new medium lymphocytes produced by large lymphocyte divisions.

It is now known that there is continuous replacement of thymic primitive cells by new cells entering the organ from the blood. This question will be discussed in the next chapter but at this point the repopulation data suggest that new cells enter the primitive thymic cell population at the rate of about 1% per day and it seems likely that these new cells enter the thymic cell system at the level of the large lymphocyte. From this data it can be deduced that large lymphocyte divisions also do not produce exactly 50% parental type and 50% daughter type offspring but tend to produce more daughter type medium lymphocytes, the deficit so produced in the large lymphocyte population being made good by the newly arrived cells seeding out from the blood.

After tritiated thymidine labelling, labelled small lymphocytes accumulate in the thymus in a linear fashion when plotted arithmetically against time. In the AKR thymus, 50% of small cells in the thymus are labelled by 1.6 days, suggesting a total population replacement time of 3—4 days. These data suggest that in the AKR thymus (and similar data have been obtained for the C57Bl thymus), small lymphocytes have a mean intrathymic life span of 3—4 days. However, the possibility exists that a small fraction of thymic lymphocytes (less than 5%) may have a longer life span, for at four days after tritiated thymidine labelling the small lymphocyte population is still only 95% labelled. From the appearance of autoradiograph sections of thymus, most of these longer-lived lymphocytes appear to reside in the medulla.

Since the size of the adult thymus remains relatively constant over long periods, it is obvious that if the total population of thymic small lymphocytes is replaced every 3—4 days, then an equal number of small lymphocytes must migrate from the organ or die locally in the organ during the same time interval. Does this cell migration or death occur on a random basis or at the end of the 3—4 days intrathymic life span?

Craddock et al. (1964) observed by chemical determinations of tritiated thymidine levels in the rat thymus that the total level of tritiated thymidine in the thymus remained remarkably constant in the first three days after labelling, after which time levels commenced falling. In contrast lymph node tritiated thymidine levels began falling immediately after labelling. We have confirmed this observation in AKR and C57Bl mice labelled with tritiated thymidine, by assessing total thymic grain counts from autoradiographs of smears of thymic lymphoid cells (Metcalf, 1965). In the interval from 1 hour to 3 days after labelling the tritiated thymidine label moved progressively from the primitive cells to the small lymphocyte population, which after day 1 came to contain the major portion of the label. Total thymic grain counts remained constant until 3 days but fell from day 4 onwards. If there had been any significant cell migration of small lymphocytes from the thymus in the 1 hour to 3 day interval after labelling, this would readily have been apparent as a fall in the total thymic grain count. Further, if one assumes that small lymphocytes are generated by the asymmetrical division of the 10% of medium lymphocytes every 8 hours as the data indicate, theoretical curves can be constructed to represent the accumulation of labelled small lymphocytes in the population, based either on the assumption of random loss or age-related loss of small lymphocytes from the thymus. The curve constructed for the random loss of labelled and unlabelled cells from the thymus in no way resembles the observed accumulation of labelled small lymphocytes in the thymus which instead almost exactly fits the theoretical curve constructed on an age-related loss basis.

It appears therefore that newly formed small lymphocytes do not migrate from, or die in, the thymus on a random basis but that most small lymphocytes migrate or die at the end of their 3—4 day intrathymic life span.

In the thymus, the primitive and mature lymphocytes are not mixed indiscriminately throughout the cortex. There are distinct zones in the cortex in which there is a high proportion of large and medium cells. These zones are situated at the outer edge of the lobule and (in thymus grafts) also along the radial vessels with their sheaths of epithelial cells. As one might expect from this, these zones also contain the greatest number of mitotic lymphocytes. Primitive cells and mitotic cells do occur throughout the remainder of the cortex but they are scattered and relatively few in number (Fig. 10).

Scattered throughout the lymphoid cells of the cortex are many reticulum cells. These are difficult to see in ordinary haematoxylin and eosin sections but are obvious in frozen sections stained to demonstrate alkaline phosphatase activity. There appears to be some heterogeneity in this population of reticulum cells either with respect to cell type or cell function at any one time. Duplicate sections stained for alkaline phosphatase, acid phosphatase, 5-esterase, 6-glucose phosphatase and adenosine triphosphatase, all reveal reticulum cells but the apparent number and distribution of positively reacting cells vary widely according to the substrate used (Metcalf and Wyllie, unpublished data). These reticulum cells are few in number compared with the lymphoid cells of the cortex and their function is little understood.

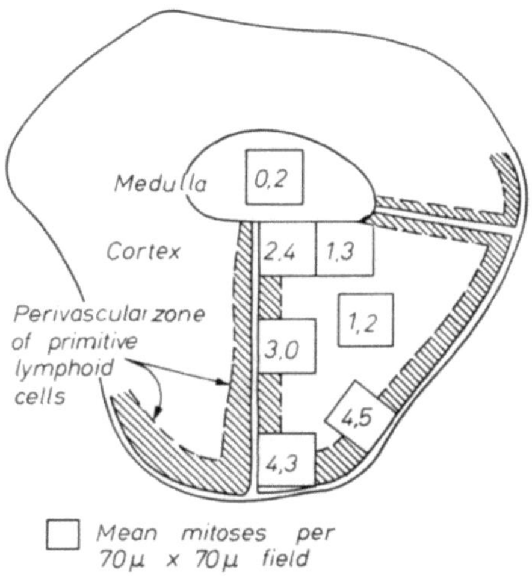

Fig. 10. Incidence of mitotic lymphocytes (mean number of mitoses in ten 70×70 μ fields) in various locations in four weeks old C57Bl subcutaneous thymus grafts

One further cell type in the thymus cortex needs some discussion. Scattered throughout the outer third of the cortex are reticulum cells having a more bulky cytoplasm than the average reticulum cell. These cells are present in the mouse thymus at all ages but the size of the cytoplasm increases progressively with age and after the age of 6 months these cells become very prominent in the thymus cortex (Metcalf and Ishidate, 1962). At this time the single oval nucleus of these cells is usually in an eccentric location and the cytoplasm is filled with granules of regular size. In haematoxylin and eosin sections, the cytoplasm is weakly eosinophilic and since the granules contain lipide, these cells have been termed "foamy cells" by some authors (Loewenthal and Smith, 1952). We have been struck by the intense positive reaction given by the granules of these cells with the Periodic Acid-Schiff reagent and have termed these cells PAS-positive reticulum cells, or PAS cells. A remarkable feature of these cells is that there is a higher incidence of mitoses in the lymphocytes in contact with these cells than in lymphocytes in adjacent areas of the cortex (Fig. 11) (Metcalf and Ishidate, 1961, 1962). Further, there is an abnormally high percentage of prophases in the PAS cell-associated lymphocyte mitoses. This association of PAS cells with lymphocyte mitoses is most evident in thymus glands in which mitotic activity is high, for example in the preleukaemic AKR thymus or in the thymus regenerating after cortisone-induced involution (Ishidate and Metcalf, 1963). The PAS cells are phagocytic and at any one time about one third of them contain pyknotic lymphocytes. Six hours after cortisone administration, virtually all the PAS cells can be shown to have phagocytosed large numbers of pyknotic lymphocytes which then are rapidly broken down. Subsequently there is an apparent increase in the granule content of the cytoplasm. The functional significance of these PAS cells is uncertain. They are actively concerned in the process of lymphocyte breakdown and may release breakdown products which become available for

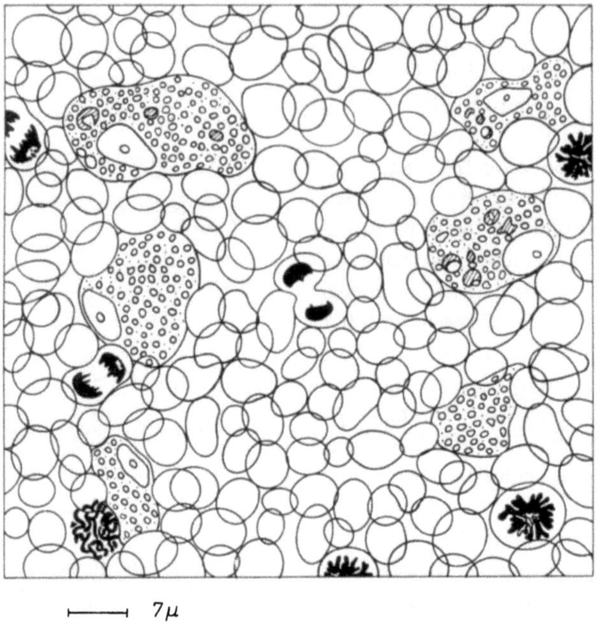

Fig. 11. Camera lucida drawing of a PAS-stained section of the thymus cortex of a 7 months old AKR mouse. Note six large reticulum cells with PAS-positive cytoplasmic granules. Three of the lymphocytes in contact with these cells are in mitosis

reutilization by other lymphoid cells. It is less certain what relation PAS cells have to lymphocyte mitotic activity, but this question will be discussed later. PAS cells are difficult to demonstrate in the thymus in other species but comparable cells probably exist in these species but may be less evident because of a less distinctive cytoplasm.

It has been suggested that the reticular epithelial cells forming sheaths around the vessels of the thymus cortex constitute a cell barrier impeding the free access of large molecules, e.g. antigens, from the blood into the thymus parenchyma. This suggestion has been made to account for the absence of lymphoid follicles and germinal centres from the thymus cortex and it has been postulated that if antigens could gain access to thymic lymphoid cells, lymphoid follicles and germinal centres would develop. In support of this suggestion, Marshall and White (1961) have shown that the direct injection of antigen into thymus tissue is followed by lymphoid follicle and germinal centre development. However, the direct injection procedure may have allowed peripheral lymphoid and macrophage cells to migrate into the thymus along the path of traumatised tissue left by the needle and these migrant cells may have been responsible for the development of the lymphoid follicles.

Systemically-administered antigens certainly are not concentrated in the adult thymus as they are in the spleen (Nossal and Mitchell, 1965) and with some antigens there is electron microscopic evidence showing what appears to be an accumulation of administered antigen in the tissue space between the radial thymic vessels and the epithelial sheaths (CLARK, 1964). However other studies have shown that at least some antigens have little difficulty in penetrating into the parenchyma of the thymus, particularly in the neonatal animal (SAINTE MARIE, 1963; GREEN and BLOCH, 1963; NOSSAL and MITCHELL, 1965). Further, the epithelial cell sheath is not complete and has large lacunae particularly in the peripheral regions of the sheath. These are large enough to allow cell passage and, as will be described later, cells regularly enter the thymus from the blood. If whole cells can enter the thymus it seems unlikely that much smaller antigen molecules would have difficulty in entering.

Recent studies on the fate of systemically-administered I^{125}-labelled Salmonella adelaide flagellar antigen have clarified the events occurring in lymphoid organs following antigen administration (NOSSAL and MITCHELL, 1965). These studies have shown that antigen readily penetrates the neonatal rat thymus parenchyma although there appears to be some impediment to antigen entry into the adult rat thymus. However it is now apparent that simple antigen penetration into an organ is not, in itself, sufficient to provoke an immune cellular response. The antigen must be trapped by a system of reticulum (macrophage) cells and concentrated in focal areas in the rudimentary lymphoid follicles before germinal centre formation is initiated (NOSSAL, ADA and AUSTIN, 1964). In the neonatal animal, these antigen trapping and concentrating macrophage cell systems are not operative and this may be the reason for the lack of immune responsiveness to such foreign antigens in the neonatal period. A somewhat similar situation exists in the adult thymus. Some of the antigen is concentrated in individual reticulum cells but there is no subsequent focalisation of antigen and indeed there may not be any follicular anlagen in the thymus cortex. Thus although antigen can enter the thymus, there is no pre-existing group of cells in the thymus which can handle the antigen and possibly there are no rudimentary follicular structures to form the framework for lymphoid follicle and germinal centre development.

In pathological states, as previously mentioned, lymphoid follicles and germinal centres can develop in the medullary areas of the thymus but the thymus medulla in many ways resembles the medullary region of lymph nodes (e.g. in its involvement in generalised reticulum cell sarcoma and its higher content of plasma cells and reticulum cells) and at least in abnormal conditions, the medulla may be equipped with cells capable of processing antigen and forming the framework for lymphoid follicles. Thus the thymus cortex appears to lack follicles and germinal centres primarily because it lacks a suitable cell system for trapping antigen and fostering the development of these structures.

Recently it was suggested that the thymus produces a factor inhibiting the initiation of primary responses to injected antigens or foreign tissue grafts (MOWBRAY, 1963). If such is the case, the thymus cortex may be capable of actively suppressing local immune responses. However these original observations have not yet been confirmed and the existence of a thymic inhibitory factor for immune responses is in some doubt at present.

Before leaving this discussion of the structure of the thymus, brief mention should be made of those agents which are known to affect the weight of the thymus. These have been reviewed ably by DOUGHERTY (1952). The thymus is extremely sensitive to a wide variety of hormonal and chemical influences. As discussed earlier, during any illness or severe stress the thymus rapidly loses weight. In fact thymus weight is the most useful practical index for assessing the amount of stress to which an animal has been subjected. It is almost certain that this effect is mediated by the action of the lymphocytolytic adrenal corticosteroids, which are secreted in increased amounts in such situations. During pregnancy and lactation the thymus also loses weight, again probably due to the increased blood levels of adrenal corticosteroids (PEPPER, 1961; ITO and HOSHINO, 1962).

The action of cortisone on the thymus has been the subject of many experimental studies (ISHIDATE and METCALF, 1963; DOUGHERTY et al., 1964). In brief, cortisone (or the active metabolite, cortisol) causes, within hours of administration, widespread death and dissolution of thymic small lymphocytes. Many of these cells are rapidly phagocytosed by local reticulum cells and PAS cells but it is suspected that many more small lymphocytes may literally disintegrate into sub microscopic fragments which are carried from the thymus in the blood stream. Because small lymphocytes make up the major portion of the thymic cell population, thymus weight rapidly falls after cortisone administration and reaches a minimum level 1—3 days after injection. Mitotic activity in large and medium lymphocytes in the thymus virtually ceases after the administration of large doses of cortisone and many of these cells are also destroyed, although they are considerably more resistant than the small lymphocytes. After the initial phase of necrosis, the thymus weight remains constant for a variable period, dependent on the dose of cortisone used. Although thymus weight remains unaltered during this period, considerable cellular reorganisation is occurring in the organ. Lymphocyte debris is rapidly removed or broken down and primitive lymphocytes again reappear in the cortex and commence mitotic activity. This mitotic activity leads to a rapid restoration of thymus weight and after a typical dose of 1 mg cortisone acetate to a young adult mouse, thymus weight is restored to pre-injection levels by day 14. The injection of ACTH produces essentially similar changes to cortisone and this hormone probably exerts its effects by stimulating the adrenals of the animal to produce excessive amounts of corticosteroids.

The thymus is more sensitive to weight loss following cortisone than either lymph nodes or spleen. It is uncertain whether this is a result of an intrinsically higher susceptibility of the thymic lymphoid cells or the fact that metabolic transformation of cortisol to inactive steroids is less rapid in the thymus than in other lymphoid tissues (DOUGHERTY et al., 1964).

The converse situation is seen in the thymus after bilateral adrenalectomy. In the mouse, thymus weight increases for several days after adrenalectomy finally reaching a new plateau. During this time mitotic activity in the primitive thymic lymphoid cells is increased (ISHIDATE and METCALF, 1963). Testosterone in large doses (5 mgm per mouse) causes thymic atrophy of a similar type to that induced by cortisone. Again the lymph nodes appear much less sensitive than the thymus and frequently the weight of the lymph nodes in testosterone-treated animals is higher than in control animals. Superficially, oestrogens have a similar action to both cortisone and testosterone, causing thymus weight loss. However the mechanism of this weight loss following oestrogen administration may differ from that of cortisone for experiments in our laboratory have indicated that the long-term administration of oestrogens can actually increase thymic mitotic indices (METCALF, unpublished data). Both testosterone and oestrogens exert a direct influence on thymus tissue and their effects are unaltered by prior adrenalectomy.

Many other agents have been shown to produce thymus weight loss e.g. irradiation, underfeeding and B vitamin deficiency, but their mechanism of action is uncertain, many probably operating via the adrenal corticosteroids. A few agents increase thymus weight, for example growth hormone and thyroid hormone (GYLLENSTEN, 1962), possibly by stimulating lymphocyte proliferation and differentiation.

It is a rather striking feature of the thymus that although the chronic application of the above agents can produce long lasting weight changes in the organ, none of these agents alters the time at which age involution occurs in the organ. This process occurs at exactly the same time as in the normal animal, the difference being merely one of the absolute weight changes involved (DOUGHERTY, 1952; ITO and HOSHINO, 1963).

Summary

The thymus is a large lymphoid organ composed of a spongework of epithelial and reticulum cells, embedded in which are dense aggregates of lymphoid cells. The organ grows rapidly in early life but has the unique feature of undergoing age involution weight loss after puberty. Its size is unaffected by antigenic stimulation but varies with the strain and sex of the animal. The lymphoid cells of the cortex exhibit intense mitotic activity but lymphoid follicles and germinal centres are absent and plasma cells are rare. Thymus lymphocyte mitotic activity is concentrated in the peripheral regions of the cortex and along the epithelial sheaths surrounding radial vessels in the cortex. Specialised reticulum cells (PAS cells) occur in the outer part of the cortex and are associated with lymphocyte mitotic activity in these regions.

The epithelial sheath cells of the thymus may constitute a partial blood/thymus barrier, blocking the penetration of antigens, but the lack of responsiveness of the thymus cortex to antigens depends primarily on the lack of suitable macrophage and other cell complexes in the cortex which are necessary for antigen handling and for providing the framework for germinal centre formation.

Many agents e.g. cortisone, testosterone and ACTH cause thymus weight loss and some e.g. growth hormone and adrenalectomy cause thymus weight increase, but these agents do not affect the occurrence or timing of thymus age involution weight loss.

Chapter 2

Thymus Grafts

The growth and repopulation of thymus grafts will be discussed in some detail as the analysis of thymus graft behaviour has given important information on the regulation of the growth and mitotic activity of thymic lymphoid tissues—information which is essential if the process of leukaemogenesis in the thymus is to be fully understood.

In the study of thymus grafts, the mouse is the animal of choice because of the availability of inbred strains which allow free transplantation of tissue or organ grafts, from one member to another of a given strain. The second advantage of the mouse lies in the fact that the mouse thymus is a relatively small organ (varying from 5—100 mgm in weight) and its blood supply needs are so small as not to require any special vascular anastomoses when grafting whole organs.

In the usual technique of grafting to the subcutaneous tissues, the intact thymus is removed from the donor under relatively aseptic conditions and immersed in a small volume of normal saline or tissue culture fluid. The recipient is anaesthetised with ether or nembutal and a small subcutaneous pocket prepared under the skin by blunt dissection with forceps. The intact thymus is then inserted gently and the skin wound closed.

An alternative site for thymus grafting which offers a number of important advantages is under the kidney capsule. In this technique, the thymus is loaded into an elongated polythene cannula which has a finely drawn out tip with a bevelled end.

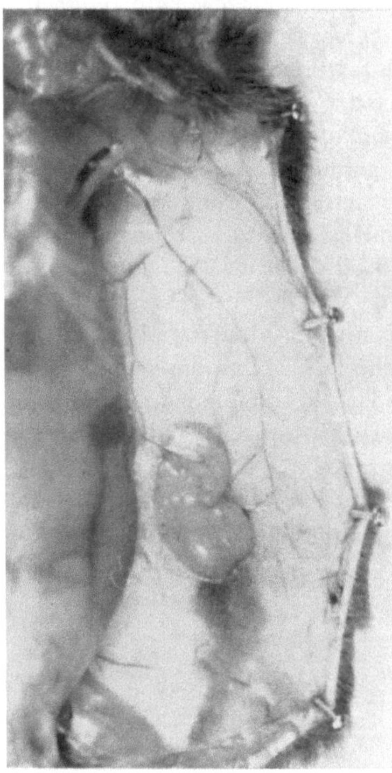

Fig. 12

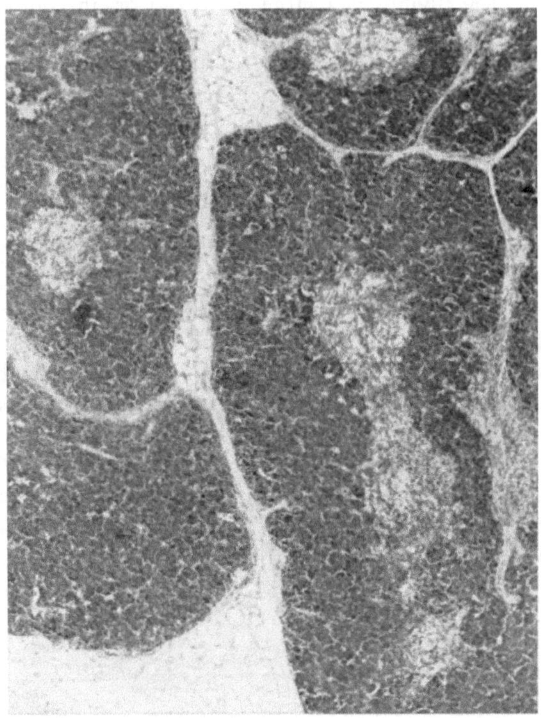

Fig. 13

Fig. 12. Thymus graft tissue in subcutaneous tissues of a C57Bl mouse. Note one vessel passing over surface of graft, but the otherwise avascular appearance

Fig. 13. Photomicrograph of section of C57Bl thymus graft tissue showing cortical and medullary areas typical of the normal thymus. H and E ×70

This cannula approximates the size of a No. 18 needle and is mounted on a syringe containing 0.5 ml of air. A small tear is made in the kidney capsule over the lower pole of the kidney and the cannula is slipped under the kidney capsule and pushed up to the upper pole of the kidney. The thymus graft is deposited in this site by gentle pressure on the syringe plunger, the accompanying air bubble being squeezed back out the hole in the kidney capsule at the lower pole.

Thymus grafts appear to take successfully in any subcutaneous site in the body. The usual sites used are over the back or the lateral and ventral aspects of the abdominal or thoracic walls. However, for special purposes, grafts may even be placed under the skin of the ear or the tail. Possibly grafts grow a little better when subcutaneous fat pads are present, for example in the axilliary or groin regions but these locations are by no means essential for successful grafting. Grafts may also be placed in the peritoneal or thoracic cavities and in the spleen.

Thymus grafts present a characteristic appearance when examined a month or more after grafting. The organ is whitish in colour and rather flat with rounded edges but still retains an obvious bi-lobed structure. Although some host blood vessels penetrate the graft capsule, these are typically very small, giving the organ a curiously avascular appearance (Fig. 12).

Histologically, thymus grafts exhibit the characteristic morphology of the normal thymus (Fig. 13). There are clearly defined medullary areas surrounded by typical dense cortical aggregates of lymphoid cells, exhibiting intense mitotic activity. As in

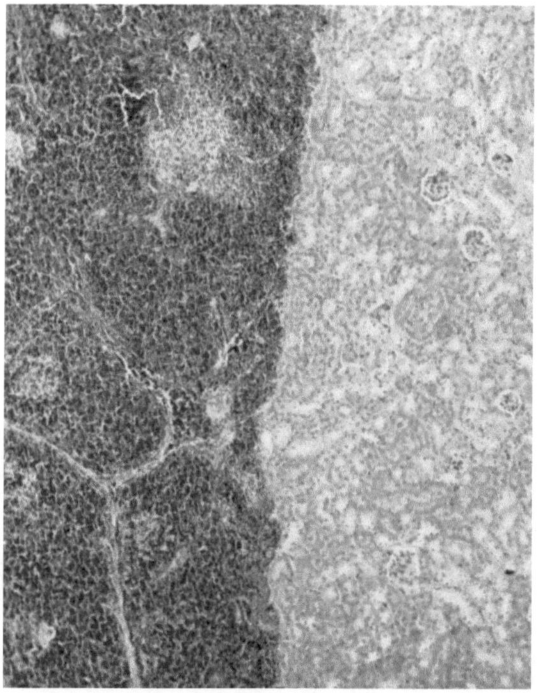

Fig. 14. Portion of a C57Bl thymus graft under the kidney capsule. Note morphology of typical thymus tissue and lack of cellular infiltration of underlying kidney tissue. H and E ×70

the normal thymus cortex, no lymphoid follicles or germinal centres are present and plasma cells are rare (less than 0.1% of thymic lymphoid cells). Cytological studies on thymus grafts have revealed (METCALF et al., 1961) that they contain the same percentage distribution of large and medium lymphocytes as the normal thymus and that these primitive cells have the same mitotic activity as the cells of the normal thymus. Autoradiographic studies on subcutaneous thymus grafts in C57Bl mice (Matsyama, Wiadrowski and Metcalf, 1966) confirmed that tritiated thymidine uptake of thymus graft cells is thymic, not lymph node in type, and that the thymus graft primitive lymphoid cells divide as rapidly as in the host thymus. The population of thymus graft small lymphocytes is replaced every three to four days as in the normal thymus. In all these respects thymus graft lymphoid cells behave in a completely different fashion from lymph node or spleen lymphoid cells.

Thymus grafts in the mouse do differ slightly from the structure of the normal mouse thymus in that the lobes tend to be broken up into large islands or lobules by stromal elements containing mesenchymal tissues and blood vessels. Almost certainly this is the result of trauma to the organ at the time of grafting, associated with the anoxic death of some thymus tissue immediately after grafting.

Grafts under the kidney capsule also exhibit the typical morphology of thymus tissue (Fig. 14). A distinct cell layer separates the thymus tissue from underlying kidney parenchymal tissue and there is no infiltration of the kidney tissue by lymphocytes from the adjacent graft. The host kidney is slightly flattened by the thymus graft, and there is a minor degree of thinning of the renal cortex adjacent to the thymus graft site but the growth and function of the grafted kidney does not differ significantly from that of the contralateral kidney.

Despite the use of isologous thymus grafts in inbred mice it is quite typical in any experiment involving large numbers of subcutaneous grafts to find that 10—15% of

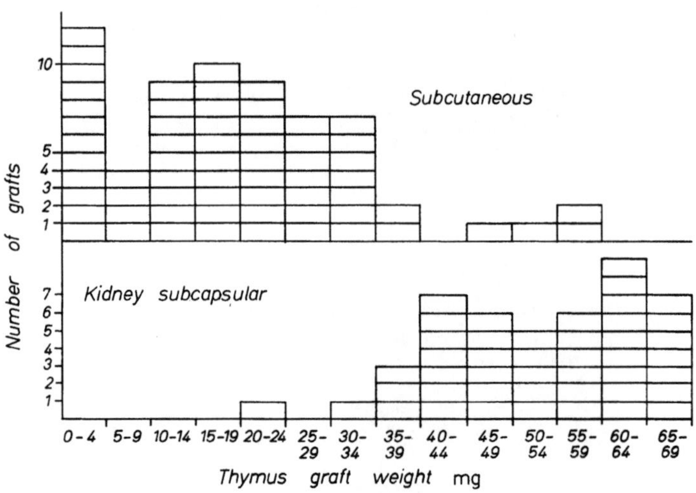

Fig. 15. Individual C57Bl thymus graft weights in (AKR×C57Bl)F_1 mice, four weeks after grafting. Weight of donor neonatal thymus at grafting, 3 mgm. Note larger and more uniform size of grafts under the kidney capsule than subcutaneous grafts

grafts fail to take. Furthermore, there is a wide variation in the maximum size attained by individual subcutaneous grafts (Fig. 15). This variability in thymus graft growth is due, almost certainly, to the variable degree of success of the grafted organ in establishing a satisfactory blood supply in the critical first few days after grafting.

Thymus grafts in the subcapsular region of the kidney are much superior in these respects. No example of failure of a graft to survive has ever been encountered by us in hundreds of such grafts and there is a much greater degree of uniformity in the size of the resulting thymus grafts (Fig. 15). Of even greater practical importance is the fact that the growth rate of grafts under the kidney capsule is three to six times that of grafts in the subcutaneous region (Fig. 16). The rate of growth of neonatal grafts under the kidney capsule even exceeds that of the normal thymus in mice of the same strain (METCALF, WAKONIG-VAARTAJA and BRADLEY, 1965).

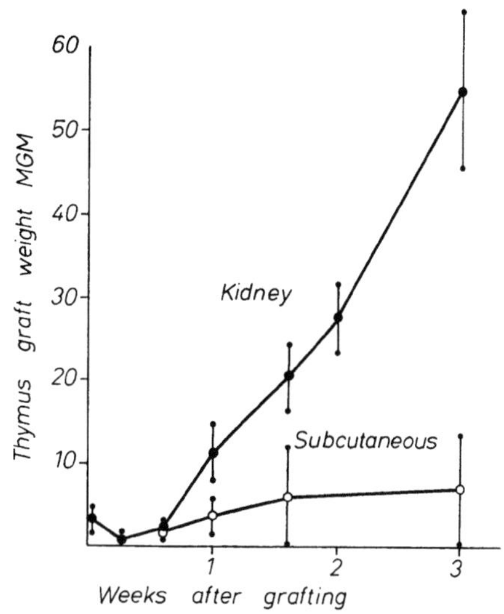

Fig. 16. Growth rates of neonatal C57Bl thymus grafts in the subcutaneous tissues and under the kidney capsule

The superior growth rate of thymus grafts under the kidney capsule appears to be the non-specific result of a better blood supply in this region rather than to any thymotropic influence from the kidney tissue. Spleen grafts in this site also exhibit a 100% success rate and a three to five times more rapid growth than in the subcutaneous tissues (METCALF and BRADLEY, 1965). Further, subcutaneous mixed organ grafts, made by mixing thymus with kidney tissue, do not exhibit any enhancement of the growth of the thymic elements of these thymus-kidney mixed grafts.

A characteristic sequence of weight changes occurs in thymus tissue following grafting, which is of special importance for understanding the regulation of thymus growth and function. When day-old thymuses are grafted to the subcutaneous tissues there is an initial weight loss due to anoxic death of much of the cortical lymphoid tissue. However after one week, the graft weight commences to increase and the graft achieves a maximum size four to six weeks after grafting. At this time further weight increase ceases and after a short period of stable weight, rapid weight loss commences, followed by a more gradual weight loss which continues for the life of the grafted animal (Fig. 17). It should be noted that the time sequence of weight changes in thymus grafts is identical with that in the normal thymus in the mouse strain used. When older mice are used as donor animals for thymus grafts, the sequence of weight changes which occurs is in conformity with what might be expected from this conclusion (METCALF et al., 1961; PEPPER, 1961 a). Thus four weeks old thymus glands, when grafted, again undergo initial necrosis and then regenerate but these grafts will never attain the maximum size of the normal thymus, for after the two to three weeks of initial necrosis, reorganisation and regeneration, the grafts are now six to seven weeks old and cannot attain a final weight greater than that of a normal six to seven week old thymus, which at that age has already begun to lose weight as a result of age involution. Similarly thymus glands from six or twelve months old donor mice can be successfully grafted to recipients of any age but the size attained will always be very small—usually smaller even than the starting weight of the thymus grafted. True "growth" of a thymus graft (that is weight increase over the weight at grafting) can only be attained when pre-involutional thymus glands are used.

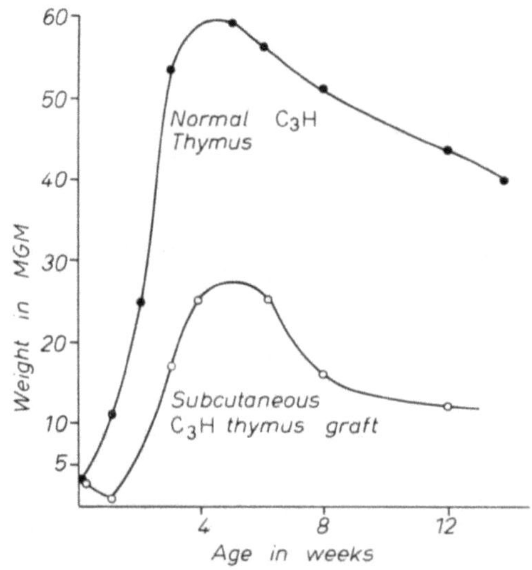

Fig. 17

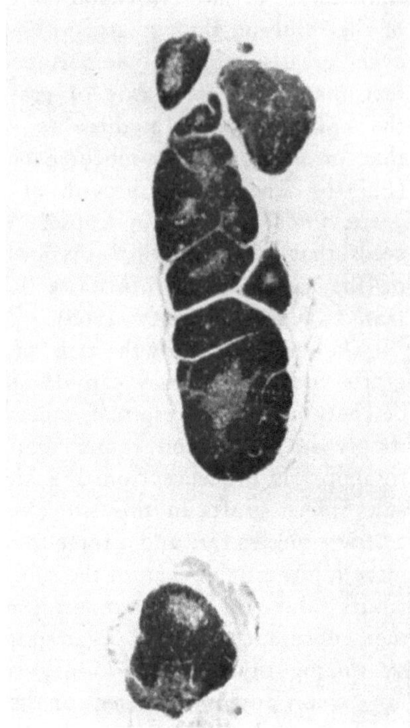

Fig. 18

Fig. 17. Weight changes with ageing in neonatal subcutaneous C3H thymus grafts, placed in six months old C3H recipients. Note that age involution weight loss in thymus grafts occurs at same age as in the normal thymus in C3H mice

Fig. 18. Section of minute thymus grafts derived from seeding of thymus fragments in the subcutaneous tissues. Note medullary tissue in each graft fragment. H and E ×22

Thymus tissue can be grafted successfully in smaller units than the whole organ or thymic lobe. Minced thymus fragments may be seeded in the subcutaneous tissues and later recovered as successful minute grafts, exhibiting typical thymic morphology. However such studies have revealed that only fragments containing medullary tissue can be successfully grafted, and each thymus fragment graft when recovered contains cortex and medulla in proportions identical with that of the normal thymus (Fig. 18) (Metcalf, 1963). When grafts were attempted using strips of thymus cortical tissue or single cell suspensions of thymus cells, no successful grafts were recovered.

A complex but very important sequence of population changes has been demonstrated to occur in the cortical lymphoid cells of thymus grafts (Metcalf and Wakonig-Vaartaja, 1964). These will be discussed in some detail because the processes they demonstrate together with recent repopulation data obtained from parabiotic animals (Harris et al., 1964) have opened up a new era in our knowledge of cellular migration streams in the normal animal of haemopoietic cells, including erythroid, myeloid and megakarocytic, as well as lymphoid cells. Our ability to follow cellular population changes in the thymus has stemmed from the introduction of the T6 marker chromosome. CBA/T6T6 mice exhibit two minute T6 marker chromosomes in every mitotic figure in the animal. When mice of this type are crossed with mice of other strains, the resulting F_1 hybrid has one such T6 marker chromosome in every mitotic cell. This F_1 hybrid can be used as a recipient for grafts of tissue from the parental strain, not carrying the T6 marker chromosome. Thus AKR thymus grafts may be placed in (AKR $\times$ T6)F_1 mice and, after the administration of colchicine to the animal, the origin of the dividing cells in the graft can be determined from the presence or absence of a T6 marker chromosome in chromosome squash preparations of the thymus graft cells.

Following the grafting of day old AKR thymus glands to adult (AKR $\times$ T6)F_1 mice, widespread death of cells (mainly lymphoid) occurs in the grafted tissues. The organ collapses inwards around surviving groups of epithelial and reticulum cells and some cortical lymphoid cells. Mitotic activity recommences in the surviving cortical lymphoid cells and there is a gradual filling out of the cortex with lymphoid cells, the vast majority of which are donor in origin (METCALF and WAKONIG-VAARAJA, 1964). This process is more obvious in grafts in the kidney subcapsular site because of the more rapid initial recovery and growth of such grafts (METCALF, WAKONIG-VAARTAJA and BRADLEY, 1965). By day 10 after grafting most thymus grafts contain a well developed lymphoid cortex which is derived almost entirely from the proliferation of cells present in the thymus at the time of grafting. There then occurs, however, a most remarkable replacement of this donor population of dividing lymphoid cells by a population of cells derived from the host. By day 21 after grafting, *all* mitoses seen in subcutaneous thymus grafts are demonstrable as being of host origin (Fig. 19). Similarly by day 30 after grafting all mitoses in kidney subcapsular grafts are of host origin. It should be emphasized that by three weeks after grafting only the lymphoid cells of the cortex continue to exhibit mitotic activity. Although donor epithelial and reticulum cells survive in thymus grafts and initially exhibit active mitosis, this mitotic activity ceases around the third week after grafting, when the thymus graft is approaching maximum size. Tritiated thymidine autoradiographic data have indicated that the population of non-dividing small lymphocytes in thymus grafts is replaced by mitotic division of the primitive cells every three to four days (MATSUYAMA, WIADROWSKI and METCALF, 1966). Thus by day 25 for subcutaneous grafts, and day 35 for kidney subcapsular grafts, it is highly probable that all lymphoid cells in thymus grafts, whether mitotic or non-mitotic, are of host origin. These findings mean that all well-established thymus grafts after four to five weeks in the recipient are permanent chimaeric organs, being composed of an epi-

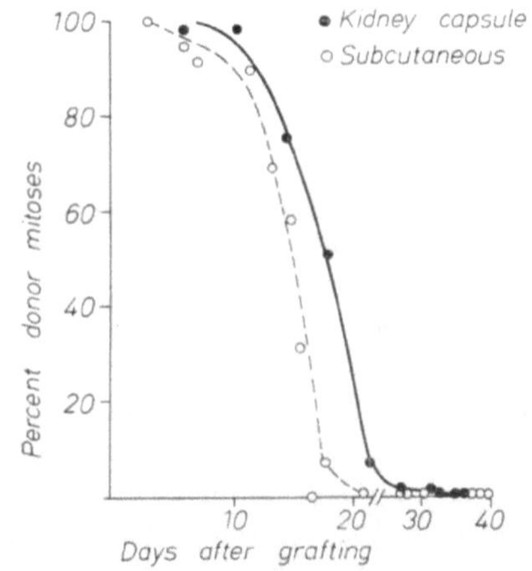

Fig. 19. Replacement of donor by host cells in AKR thymus grafts in the subcutaneous tissues or under the kidney capsule of (AKR$\times T_6$)F_1 hosts. Data from 146 subcutaneous grafts and 22 kidney capsule grafts

thelial and reticulum cell spongework of *donor* origin, embedded in the interstices of which are dense aggregates of proliferating lymphoid cells of *host* origin. Such thymus grafts are ideal for determining which of the two cell systems is responsible for specific behaviour patterns of cells in the thymus e.g. the rate of thymic lymphocyte proliferation or the susceptibility to neoplasia development of thymic lymphoid cells.

Neither thymectomy nor irradiation of the host animal, nor the use of adult rather than neonatal donor thymic tissue affects the rate, or completeness, of this population replacement of thymus graft lymphoid cells by host cells.

It may be wondered whether this host cell replacement of thymus graft cells is unique for thymus grafts. Parallel experiments with whole spleen grafts have indicated that a similar cell replacement process occurs in such grafts but at a slightly slower rate than for thymus grafts. By day 35 after grafting all mitotic cells in subcutaneous spleen grafts can be shown to be of host origin (METCALF and WAKONIG-VAARTAJA, 1964 a). With mouse spleen tissue, however, host cell repopulation is not limited to lymphoid cells, for mitotically active populations of erythroid, myeloid and megakarocytic cells occur in the mouse spleen and the data therefore indicate that replacement also occurs of these other cell types.

Confirmatory evidence of host cell repopulation of thymus and spleen grafts was obtained by GREEN (1964) who showed the presence of F_1 cells in parental thymus and spleen grafts in F_1 mice by testing the ability of cell suspensions from these grafts to induce runting in test animals, and by *in vitro* cytotoxic tests.

Although the nature of these thymus graft experiments allows only one population exchange to be observed, the data suggest that this process may occur repetetively—in other words there may be a continuous replacement of thymic lymphoid stem cells by blood-borne cells from elsewhere in the animal.

Does this data from thymus grafts give a true indication of events occurring in the normal thymus? In an elegant series of experiments, HARRIS and co-workers (1964) studied mitotic populations in the thymus, spleen, lymph nodes and bone marrow of pairs of CBA and CBA/T6T6 mice united in parabiosis. The data clearly indicated that over a period of two months after union the mitotic populations in the spleen and lymph nodes of each partner came to contain approximately 50% of mitotic cells derived from other partner. This indicates that probably all primitive cells capable of division in these organs were replaced by blood-borne cells during that period. After the mice were separated from parabiotic union, the mitotic populations tended to revert to host cell type over a further period of about two months (FORD, personal communication). These data indicate that complete and continuous replacement of the stem cells in the spleen and lymph nodes by cells entering the organs from the blood, occurs about every two months during normal life. The data for thymic cells indicated a similar replacement process but unlike the data from thymus grafts, indicated that the replacement process, although continuous, may not be complete. Possibly 25% of mitotic cells in the normal thymus may not be replaced by blood-borne cells and these may be permanently self-reproducing or more likely, replaced by the endogenous generation of new stem cells either by the division of thymic epithelial cells (as is postulated by AUERBACH, 1961, to occur during embryogenesis) or by the dedifferentiation of thymic small lymphocytes to primitive cells (possibly c.f. the behaviour of small lymphocytes *in vitro* after exposure to phytohaemagglutinin).

The reversal of the chimaeric state in parabiotic CBA/CBAT6T6 mice following breakage of the union suggests that primitive cells do not simply recirculate from one organ to another. Instead it seems likely that new potential stem cells are continually being produced in the body and being distributed to the various haemopoietic organs via the blood. The parabiosis experiments do not establish precisely the origin of these cells but since the bone marrow shows only minimal replacement of dividing cells by cells of haematogenous origin, the bone marrow seems the most likely source of repopulating stem cells. This conclusion is supported by studies on the capacity of cell suspensions of various organs to repopulate the haemopoietic organs of lethally irradiated recipients (FORD and MICKLEM, 1963). Spleen and bone marrow cells were able to repopulate all organs but thymus and lymph node cell suspensions were able only to repopulate lymph node tissue and not bone marrow or thymus. Since the supply of potential stem cells is not significantly depleted by splenectomy and since the normal spleen is continuously repopulated, whereas the bone marrow is not, this suggests that the bone marrow is the primary source of stem cells and that the spleen serves as a second level reservoir of such cells.

The morphological appearance of the circulating cells repopulating the haemopoietic organs has not been established with certainty but it appears probable that these cells have the morphology of small lymphocytes, regardless of their ultimate fate—that is regardless of whether they are destined to become primitive lymphoid, erythroid or myeloid cells (CUDKOWICZ et al., 1964).

This new body of knowledge on the existence of migration streams of haemopoietic stem cells and the continuous repopulation of haemopoietic organs is of obvious importance for many aspects of haematology. In the context of the thymus, these processes need to be kept in mind when considering the regulation of thymic lymphopoiesis and the origin of the neoplastic cells in thymic lymphoma development, questions which shall be returned to later.

As described earlier, neonatal thymus grafts undergo a series of weight changes which reproduce the age-related weight changes occurring in the normal thymus. The growth achieved by a thymus graft is determined by the age of the thymus when grafted and is largely independent of the age of the recipient (METCALF et al., 1961). Similarly the size attained by a thymus graft is not affected by thymectomy of the recipient.

Even more striking is the observation that when more than one thymus is grafted to a single recipient, each thymus graft attains the same size it would have if grafted alone (METCALF, 1963). In our experience we have encountered no limit in the number of thymus glands (50 or more) which may be grafted to a single recipient. Even multiple grafts in hugh conglomerates in the subcutaneous tissue all appear to grow and function perfectly. The capacity of multiple thymus grafts to grow to full size and exhibit full mitotic activity—that is to grow in an autonomous fashion—in normal animals appears to be unique amongst normal tissues and offers an unrivalled opportunity for studying both the effects of various agents on thymus tissue in readily accessible sites, and the effects of thymus tissue, in virtually unlimited amounts, on various functions of the host animal ("?hyperthymic state").

As referred to above, thymus tissue can be minced into small fragments and grafted successfully in a single subcutaneous pocket. We have carried out many experiments in which mixed minces of thymus with other tissues have been grafted to recipient mice. Spleen fragments, mixed with thymus fragments before grafting, form striking mosaic organs of alternating red spleen tissue and white thymus tissue (Fig. 20). There is little evidence of cell migration from one type of tissue to the other

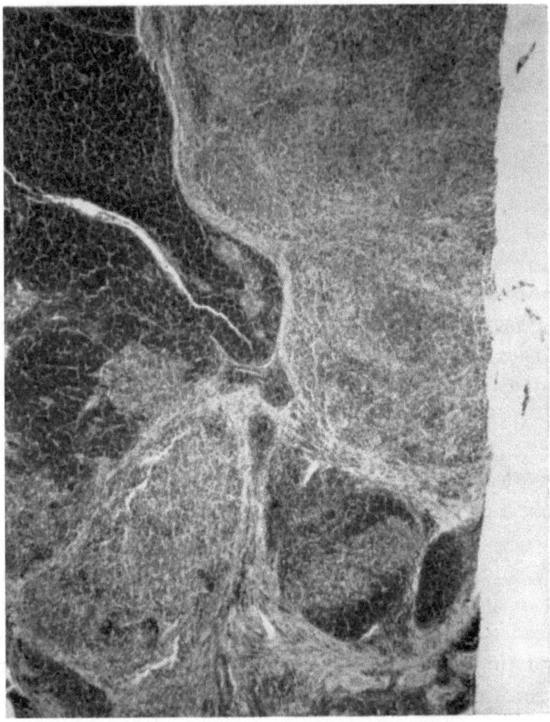

Fig. 20. Portion of a mixed organ graft of C57Bl thymus and spleen tissue. Note lighter spleen areas with lymphoid follicles and darker areas of thymus cortical lymphoid tissue. H and E ×60

although the spleen components of such mixed grafts attain a larger size than when grafted alone (METCALF, 1964 a). No lymphoid follicles or germinal centres are found in the thymus cortical regions of such mixed grafts even though active germinal centres may be present in the spleen lymphoid follicles adjacent to this tissue.

Thymus fragments may also be grafted successfully in combination with fragments of lung, kidney, liver, salivary gland, brain and a number of other tissues. Such mixed organ grafts should have many interesting uses in studies of tissue interactions between the thymus and other tissues.

It has been claimed that thymus grafts differ from the normal thymus in being able to develop lymphoid follicles, germinal centres and plasma cells, when the host is antigenically stimulated (STUTMAN and ZINGALE, 1964). Rats bearing subcutaneous thymus grafts were injected with diphtheria toxoid—antigen being injected subcutaneously in the region of the grafts. The authors reported that two weeks after the last antigen injection, lymphoid follicles and germinal centres were present in the cortical regions of the grafts and that as many as 24% of the thymus graft cells were members of the plasma cell series. We have attempted to repeat these observations with thymus grafts in mice, using the same dosage schedule of the antigen, but were unable to confirm these findings. At no time did thymus graft plasma cells exceed 0.1% (the percentage of plasma cells found in the normal thymus). Similarly thymus grafts placed in the beds of resected lymph nodes or intrasplenically, adjacent to spleen lymphoid follicles, showed no excessive numbers of plasma cells and no lymphoid follicles or germinal centres.

However, in one respect, thymus grafts do appear to behave in a manner unlike that of the normal thymus. It is characteristic in many species, during pregnancy and lactation, that the thymus undergoes severe weight loss, due to cellular depletion of the lymphoid cortex (PEPPER, 1961; ITO and HOSHINO, 1962). This phenomenon is mediated almost certainly by the elevated levels of lymphocytolytic adrenal corticosteroids circulating during pregnancy and lactation. Although thymus grafts do show a slight weight loss during pregnancy of the host, they appear to be significantly less severely affected than the host thymus (METCALF, 1964 c). A similar quantitative difference has been observed between the response of the normal thymus and thymus grafts to the injection of testosterone—again more severe weight loss occurs in the normal thymus than in thymus grafts. In both situations thymus grafts more closely resemble lymph nodes in their reactivity to these agents than thymus tissue. However as described earlier, the pattern of lymphopoiesis in thymus grafts is clearly thymic, not lymph node, in type and the basis for this somewhat different sensitivity of thymus graft tissue to pregnancy and testosterone remains to be established.

Summary

Whole organ thymus grafts or thymus fragment grafts may be made successfully in almost any site in the body, provided thymic medullary tissue is included in the tissue grafted. The kidney subcapsular site is clearly superior to the usual subcutaneous site for such grafts. All thymus grafts become repopulated by host lymphoid cells and are thus chimaeric organs, composed of donor epithelial and reticulum cells and host lymphoid cells. Thymus grafts undergo age involution weight changes based on the age of the graft and unrelated to the age of the host. The size attained by thymus grafts is unaffected by thymectomy of the host or by the presence of other thymus grafts in the same animal. Mixed organ grafts can be created by grafting mixtures of thymus fragments with other tissue fragments.

Chapter 3

Lymphocyte Migration from the Thymus

In an animal like the mouse it is relatively simple to calculate from the weights of the various lymphoid organs and the mitotic indices of the lymphoid cells in these organs that the thymus is the major production site of lymphocytes in the body. Thus in adult six months old C3H and AKR mice, the thymus probably produces between 40 and 65 percent of all new lymphocytes (Table 2) (METCALF and NAKAMURA, 1962). This conclusion is reinforced by the tritiated thymidine autoradiographic data discussed earlier which showed that the rate of replacement of the small lymphocyte population in the thymus far exceeds that in lymph nodes, blood or bone marrow. Calculations on the situation in humans are more difficult because of incomplete data but it is likely that in children at least a very similar situation exists to that found in the mouse.

Table 2. *Comparison of Lymphocyte Production in Various Lymphoid Organs in Six Months Old Male C3H and AKR Mice*

Organ	Mean weight mg		Mean number of mitoses per 1000 cells		Percent of total body lymphocyte production	
	C3H	AKR	C3H	AKR	C3H	AKR
Thymus	32	50	4.1	7.0	40%	66%
Subcutaneous lymph nodes	95	83	0.4	0.6	12%	9%
Mesenteric node	32	34	1.5	1.8	15%	12%
Spleen (lymphoid follicles)	30	25	0.4	0.6	4%	3%
Peyer's patches	38	33	2.6	1.6	29%	10%

Since the weight of the thymus remains relatively constant over long intervals, new cell formation in this organ must be balanced by an equivalent amount of cell death or migration from the organ. Although pyknotic cells are common in the normal thymus even during the phase of active growth in early life (METCALF, 1964), it seems to have been tacitly assumed by most that thymus weight is kept constant by a massive export of lymphocytes from the thymus to the rest of the body—primarily to the non-thymic lymphoid organs.

In support of this concept many experiments have been made to determine the fate of suspensions of labelled thymic lymphocytes when injected intravenously into various species. This work has been reviewed by FICHTELIUS (1960). In general, injected thymic lymphoid cells have been shown to seed in the liver and spleen of normal animals. In lethally irradiated animals, thymic cells have been shown to seed and proliferate in the lymph nodes but not in the thymus. In this latter type of animal thymic cells were found not to be able to give rise to cells of either the erythroid or myeloid series.

Certainly these thymus cell injection studies have demonstrated the capacity of thymic cells to "home" in host lymphoid organs and under certain conditions to proliferate in these organs—but do these experiments really prove that thymic lymphocytes normally leave the thymus in large numbers? Cell injection studies naturally involve a considerable degree of manipulation of these cells *in vitro* and this may well affect their physiological state and subsequent behaviour on reinjection. Of more importance is the doubtful thesis on which such experiments are based. Presumably if one made with care a single cell suspension of liver cells and injected them intravenously into a recipient one could show that many liver cells would lodge in various tissues and possibly that some would survive and under some circumstances even proliferate. However, no-one would conclude from such an experiment that liver cells were normally exported to other organs via the blood. Do the thymic cell injection studies really indicate any more than this hypothetical liver cell experiment? It is true that thymic lymphocytes are freely motile cells, of a type accustomed to passage in and out of blood vessels (MARCHESI and GOWANS, 1964), and it is not unreasonable to expect that occasionally such cells in the thymus may enter the general circulation—but do *all* thymic cells migrate from the organ every three to four days, as required by the autoradiographic data?

The question of whether or not lymphoid cells leave the thymus could be answered readily enough if some method could be found for labelling thymic lymphoid cells without labelling other body lymphoid cells. This has not yet been achieved by any systemically administered label but recently two attempts have been made to label the guinea pig thymus (suitable because of its subcutaneous cervical location) by the direct intraorgan injection of tritiated thymidine (NOSSAL, 1964; MURRAY and WOODS, 1964). These injections were carried out in such a manner as to minimise spillover of isotope into the animal. In both investigations, in the days following labelling, heavily labelled lymphoid cells (presumably thymic in origin) were observed in the spleen and lymph nodes, particularly in newborn animals. However in the better controlled work of NOSSAL, the number of thymus "migrants" was surprisingly small in relation to the production rate of thymic cells. Certain technical objections can be raised to these experiments, namely that spillage of label was not completely prevented, that direct labelling of some blood lymphocytes is known to occur, and that some destruction of intra-thymic architecture was inevitably produced by the injection procedure. Despite these objections it seems fair to concur with the authors that these experiments indicate that some thymic cells do leave the organ and seed in peripheral lymphoid organs. The same experiments suggest however that possibly the majority of the lymphoid cells produced in the thymus may remain in this organ.

We have attempted to answer this question of cell migration from the thymus by studying the labelling patterns of lymphoid cells in C57Bl mice carrying multiple thymus grafts (MATSUYAMA, WIADROWSKI and METCALF, 1966). In these studies two months old C57Bl mice were grafted subcutaneously with 12 to 48 one day old C57Bl thymus glands and one month after grafting the mice, along with control mice, were given a single intravenous injection of 5 μCi/gm of tritiated thymidine. At the time of isotopic labelling the mice carried 250—1150 mgm of thymus graft tissue in addition to their own thymus (50 mgm) and the weight of their non-thymic lymphoid organs totalled approximately 250 mgm. It was shown that the thymus graft labelling pattern was identical with that of the host thymus and control thymuses—thus by day 3 after labelling up to 90% of the graft lymphoid cells were labelled. At this time only 10% of the host lymph node or blood lymphocytes were labelled. Mice of this type were followed until day 14 after labelling but at no time did the percentage of labelled lymphocytes in the lymph nodes or blood of grafted mice rise above control levels. If cell migration occurs from the thymus tissue to make way for newly formed small lymphocytes, then the 90% labelled population present at day 3 must leave the thymus tissue between days 3—8, that is within the next thymic cycle. With the techniques used, as small an increment as 2% in the population of labelled lymphocytes in the lymph nodes or blood could have been detected. No such increment was observed, and calculations from the relative weights of thymus tissue and host non-thymic lymphoid tissues indicated that fewer than 0.5% of cells produced in the thymus grafts or host thymus could have seeded in the host lymphoid tissues during the observation period. Observations on the liver, kidney and gut of these thymus grafted animals also failed to reveal any excessive accumulation of labelled lymphoid cells in these organs. It has been concluded from these studies that very few lymphocytes produced in the thymus ever leave the organ.

It might be argued that an animal carrying multiple thymus grafts has some special mechanism for preventing the escape of these excess lymphocytes from the grafts. This may be so, but since the labelling patterns in thymus grafts were identical with those in the normal thymus and since no excess numbers of pyknotic cells were observed in such thymus grafts, this argument requires the existence of an effective mechanism for destroying small lymphocytes in the thymus every three to four days, but giving little visible evidence of its existence. This conclusion seems equally applicable to the normal thymus.

From the above considerations it seems likely that relatively few cells produced in the thymus ever leave the organ, the vast majority being destroyed on a non-random basis at the end of three to four days.

Despite the fact that few thymic cells leave the organ it should not be concluded that such limited cell migration as does occur is necessarily of little importance to the body. It is quite clear from the data described earlier that the average life span of non-thymic lymphocytes is much longer than that of thymic lymphocytes (possibly 30—100 days versus 3 days). Even a small percentage of cells migrating from the thymus could be a valuable source of new cells for these tissues and on this basis alone thymectomy might be expected to lead to a slow decrease in nonthymic lymphoid organ weights.

Reif and Allen (1964) have reported that AKR thymic lymphoid cells contain a specific antigen. They reported the presence of a small percentage of cells with this antigen in populations of AKR spleen and lymph node cells and have suggested that this is evidence of migration of lymphocytes from the thymus to the non-thymic lymphoid organs. Such claims need to be supported by studies on the effect of thymectomy on this lymph node cell population, since it could be argued that the different antigenicity merely resulted from different physiological states of lymphoid cells at the time of testing and that a true heterogeneity exists in local lymph node populations with respect to this physiological state. However even if this antigenic evidence does indicate thymus cell migration, this thymic cell content of lymph nodes and spleen could be built up by cell migration from the thymus, of the magnitude envisaged in the present discussion (that is, less than 1% of the daily cell production). It is possible for a significant percentage of the lymph node cells to become derived from this small number of migrating thymic cells if the migratory thymic cells live much longer than the average lymph node cell, or if the population size of these migrants is built up by clonal proliferation following stimulation by an antigen to which the other lymphoid cells in the lymph node do not respond. In both situations, beginning with a very small number of migrant cells, it is quite possible to envisage a build-up in the population of these cells to such a degree that they might come to be a major fraction of the cell population.

It should be re-emphasized that thymic and lymph node lymphocytes differ not only in size but also in heterogeneity of cell size. If large scale migration of thymic lymphoid cells to the lymph nodes is postulated, then it must also be postulated that these cells become radically altered in size once they seed in the lymph nodes. This process may well occur, but would fit more readily a situation where small numbers of thymus migrants were entering the lymph nodes rather than a situation where massive numbers of thymic cells were arriving daily in the lymph nodes.

The failure of thymectomy to have any effect for several weeks on lymph node size or cellularity (see later) also argues against a continuous mass influx of lymphocytes into the lymph nodes from the thymus.

Certain data appear to contradict the conclusion that few of the cells produced in the thymus leave the organ. A number of investigators have shown in chromosome marker experiments that thymus-grafted, thymectomised mice contain a high proportion of mitotic cells of graft origin in host lymph nodes (HARRIS and FORD, 1964; LEUCHARS, CROSS and DAVIES, 1964; MILLER, 1965). This is certainly indisputable evidence for a substantial migration of thymus graft cells into the host. However these observations have not established the time at which this cell migration from the graft occurred. The thymus graft is commonly mechanically disrupted during the grafting process. Further it is now well known that substantial necrosis of thymus tissue occurs immediately after grafting and this is accompanied by a widespread breakdown of the architectural framework of this tissue. During the immediate post-grafting period it is possible that many cells may escape from the disrupted graft tissue, lodge in host organs and subsequently proliferate freely—particularly if the host is in a lymphocyte-depleted state. However such cell migration may no longer occur once the architecture of the thymus grafts is restored. Even the double thymus grafting type of experiment carried out by HARIS and FORD (1964), where a thymus graft is taken from the original recipient and placed in a second recipient (again seeding cells to the recipient's lymph nodes) does not eliminate the possibility that migration of cells from the grafts is confined to the first few days after grafting.

The tritiated thymidine data from the multiple thymus-grafted mice described above come from animals in which the thymus grafts were fully regenerated before tests were applied for cell migration, and in this situation (more nearly related to the functional state of the normal thymus) no such large scale migration was demonstrated.

It is frequently stated in the literature that cortisone leads to weight loss in the thymus by causing lymphocytes to emigrate from the thymus. This thesis seems also to be advanced to cover stressful situations during infections and is used in support of the idea that in such situations the thymus exports large numbers of antigenically competent cells to the lymph nodes to be used for defence purposes. We have made direct observations on this alleged occurrence in multiple thymus-grafted animals which had been given a large dose of cortisone (MATSUYAMA and METCALF, unpublished data). Three months old C57Bl mice carrying 250 mgm of thymus graft tissue were labelled with tritiated thymidine. Three days later, observations on control mice showed that up to 90% of thymus and thymus graft lymphocytes were labelled. These animals were then injected subcutaneously with 2 mgm of cortisone acetate and the blood was examined at intervals from 0—24 hours to determine the total number of lymphocytes and the percentage of labelled lymphocytes. All mice were killed and examined 24 hours after cortisone administration. At this time thymus graft weights were only 100 mgm—that is an average of 150 mgm of labelled thymus graft tissue had been lost over the 24 hour observation period. The analysis of blood lymphocytes showed that the total lymphocytes fell to 1,000 per mm^3 by

6 hours after cortisone and remained at this level throughout 24-hour observation period. The percentage of labelled lymphocytes in the blood at no time rose above control levels of 10% in C57Bl mice not injected with cortisone. If lymphocytes migrated from thymus tissue under the influence of cortisone it can be calculated from the data how long each of the lymphocytes could spend in the blood, in transit from the thymus tissue, and not cause any detectable rise in the total number of lymphocytes or the percentage labelling of blood lymphocytes. In the data from the multiple thymus-grafted mice, this figure approximates ten seconds—an improbably short period. It seems likely therefore that the vast majority of thymic lymphocytes do not leave the organ after cortisone administration, and since thymus tissue weight does decrease sharply there must be massive local death of cells to account for this weight loss. Such *in situ* death of thymic lymphocytes following cortisone administration is of course well known and has been documented repeatedly (DOUGHERTY et al., 1964). In essence then, all cortisone administration or stress appears to do is to accelerate the normal process of intra-thymic destruction of small lymphocytes. It seems unlikely therefore, during the stress of infections or the mild stress of antigen administration, that there is any substantial excess migration of potentially useful lymphoid cells from the thymus to locally reacting lymphoid organs.

If most thymic lymphocytes do not leave the thymus, and yet whilst in the thymus exhibit little morphological evidence of any functional activity, one might legitimately raise the question of the purpose of the intense lymphopoiesis occurring in the thymus. This is still one of the major unsolved problems of the thymus.

Summary

There is evidence that some lymphocytes produced in the thymus migrate from this organ to other lymphoid organs. However the vast majority (99%) of cells produced in the thymus in the normal animal appear to die locally in the thymus at the end of their intrathymic life span of three to four days.

Chapter 4

Regulation of Thymic Lymphopoiesis

Lymphopoiesis is extremely active in the thymus. The primitive thymic lymphoid cells probably divide more frequently than any other cell type in the adult animal (every 6—8 hours) and even the non-dividing population of small lymphocytes in the thymus is replaced at a remarkably rapid rate (every 3—4 days). This spectacular lymphopoietic activity implies the operation of an intense proliferative stimulus on thymic lymphoid cells. Further, since thymic lymphopoiesis differs so obviously from that in other lymphoid organs, it suggests that this proliferative stimulus either has a selective effect on thymic cells, or more likely, has an intrinsic origin with the organ itself.

It may be argued that in the thymus, lymphoid cells are merely allowed to give free expression to their inherent capacity to proliferate, rather than that they are subjected to a true proliferative stimulus. This is probably only a question of semantics since it is likely that all "proliferative" stimuli merely represent various types of removal of cells from the inhibition of proliferation associated with cellular differentiation and tissue interactions. As was mentioned earlier, the non-thymic lymphoid tissues require antigenic stimulation before being able to exhibit maximum proliferative activity. The proliferative activity of normal thymic lymphoid cells is at least equal to, and usually exceeds, that of antigenically-stimulated non-thymic lymphoid cells. Since antigenic stimulation appears not to be involved in the regulation of proliferation in the thymus, this logically requires the existence of an alternative proliferative stimulus for thymic lymphoid cells.

Three distinct factors need consideration in analysing the regulation of thymic lymphopoiesis: 1. the nature and supply of the incoming repopulating cells for the thymus, 2. the nature of the general hormonal environment of the animal, and 3. the nature of the intrinsic thymic factors stimulating lymphopoiesis.

1. The Nature and Supply of Incoming Repopulating Cells for the Thymus

Like the situation in the spleen and lymph nodes, lymphopoiesis in the thymus is dependent on the availability and the nature of the new blood-borne cells entering the organ to replace the existing primitive cells. If this supply of new cells were to be curtailed or the cells themselves were to become altered, then changes would probably occur either in the size of the thymus or the rate of proliferation of the thymic lymphoid cells.

The thymus decreases in size and proliferative activity with increasing age of the animal. Is this the result of a decreased supply of new stem cells? This question has been investigated in our laboratory by testing the growth capacity of neonatal thymus grafts in very old animals (METCALF, 1965 a). Since thymus grafts are known to be repopulated by host cells, any decrease in the supply of thymus repopulating cells in the old animal should make itself evident as a decreased growth capacity of such thymus grafts, particularly if more than one graft is placed in the same host animal.

Table 3. *Weights Attained by Multiple Whole C57Bl Thymus Grafts Four Weeks after Grafting to Young and Old C57Bl Mice*

Age of recipient at grafting	Number of thymus glands grafted per recipient [1]	Number of recipients	Mean host thymus weight mgm	Mean total thymus graft weight per recipient mgm	Mean weight of individual thymus grafts mgm
2 months	1	28	47	24	24
	12	41	42	262	22
	24	2	48	609	25
	48	2	36	1160	24
20 months	12	18	16	185	16
	24	2	15	467	19

[1] Mean weight of each donor thymus gland = 3 mgm.

In our experiments, twelve or twenty-four 1-day old C57Bl thymus glands were grafted subcutaneously to each 19—20 months old C57Bl recipient and the size of the grafts determined 4 weeks later. The data (Table 3) suggested that there was some limitation of the total mass of thymus graft tissue achieved in the old hosts compared with that in young adult hosts. However, despite this limitation, the total mass of thymus graft tissue achieved far exceeded the weight of the host thymus or even the maximum weight of the thymus (60 mgm) in early life in C57Bl mice. It seems therefore that the available number of cells capable of repopulating thymus tissue may decline in old age but it is still far in excess of that required for maintenance of the normal thymus at its maximum size. Thus a shortage of repopulating cells in old age does not seem to be a significant factor in determining weight loss in the thymus with advancing age.

Histological examination of neonatal thymus grafts in old hosts revealed no obvious difference in the incidence or distribution of mitotic lymphoid cells in the graft cortical tissue compared with similar grafts in young hosts. This suggests that those old host cells which did repopulate the thymus grafts were able to proliferate as rapidly as younger repopulating cells. Thus there also was no evidence of any intracellular ageing process in the repopulating cells themselves, which prevents them from proliferating freely when stimulated.

In various experimental situations a shortage of thymus repopulating cells may be of greater importance than in the ageing situation. Thus normal young thymus grafts placed in animals previously exposed to whole body irradiation do not grow as well as in normal hosts and display evidence of a decreased rate of repopulation and of difficulty in proliferation of the cells which do enter the grafts (Carnes and Kaplan, 1956). This is due probably in part at least to the irradiation having destroyed or damaged cells which could have repopulated the graft, since the intravenous injection of normal bone marrow cells restores normal graft growth and morphology in irradiated hosts. It is possible that chemical carcinogens, leukaemia viruses and hormonal agents such as testosterone may also influence either the number or the nature of the cells repopulating thymus tissue. A similar situation could be anticipated in diseases of the tissues (probably the bone marrow) supplying the repopulating stem cells.

2. Nature of the General Hormonal Environment of the Animal

As previously mentioned many hormones affect the rate of proliferation of thymic lymphoid cells and the total thymus mass. The most active group in this regard are the lymphocytolytic adrenal corticosteroids. Even physiological levels of these hormones can be demonstrated to have a suppressive effect on thymic lymphopoiesis and removal of the adrenals leads to an immediate increase in thymic lymphocyte proliferative activity and in thymus size (Ishidate and Metcalf, 1963; Dougherty et al., 1964).

The adrenal steroids represent the major inhibitory system in the body dampening down lymphocyte proliferation in the thymus. In strains of mice such as the AKR where adrenal function is subnormal, it may be demonstrated that the thymus is larger and more active mitotically than in other strains. In part at least these differences are due to the subnormal functioning of the adrenal in AKR mice (Metcalf, 1960 a).

It is likely that many factors producing thymus atrophy operate by stimulating an increased production of adrenal steroids. Thus in mice operative stress, fighting, overcrowding and infections probably all produce thymus atrophy via this system.

The sex steroids—oestrogens, and particularly testosterone—also cause thymus weight loss and affect thymic lymphocyte proliferation. Their mode of action is uncertain but they appear equally effective in the absence of the adrenals, suggesting that whatever their mechanism of action, it probably does not involve the adrenal cortex.

Under-nutrition and B vitamin deficiencies reduce thymus weight and lymphopoiesis but it seems probable that this is the direct result of inadequate nutrition of the thymic lymphoid cells themselves, preventing them from synthesising cellular material at maximum rates thus reducing the rate of subsequent cell division. Malnutrition may have a direct toxic effect on lymphoid cells, but this is less certain.

A few factors appear to increase the size of the thymus although their effect on actual proliferation of thymic lymphoid cells has not been documented. Thus the administration of growth hormone and possibly thyroid hormone (HOHN, 1959) leads to thymus weight increase. It is uncertain what mechanisms are involved and whether or not adrenal cortex function is modified by these agents.

In general terms then, most systemic body influences tend to be suppressive for thymic lymphopoiesis and this very fact reinforces the earlier conclusion that there must be a powerful local proliferative influence in the thymus to balance these general inhibitory influences.

Are changes in these general hormonal and nutritional influences in the animal responsible for any of the characteristics of thymic lymphopoiesis—particularly age involution? When neonatal C3H thymus grafts were placed in 6 months old, post-involutional, C3H hosts, active growth of the thymus grafts occurred during the same period as the host thymus was losing weight (METCALF et al., 1961). This would suggest that the normal systemically circulating inhibitory influences in a middle aged animal are not inimical for active thymus growth. In female AKR mice, age involution is delayed long enough to make feasible a study of thymus graft growth in pre-involutional hosts. A comparison of the growth of neonatal AKR grafts in 4 weeks old (pre-involutional) and 3 months old (post-involutional) AKR mice indicated that grafts attained a slightly larger size in pre-involutional than in post-involutional hosts (METCALF et al., 1961). This finding would suggest that general inhibitory influences (if they are increased in the post-involutional host) may suppress, to a minor degree, thymus graft growth and thymic lymphoid mitotic activity. However it is possible that the supply of repopulating thymic stem cells may be greater in the pre-involutional animal than in the post-involutional host. At all events the differences involved in thymus graft growth in the two types of host were minor. When the growth was studied of whole neonatal C57Bl thymus glands placed under the kidney capsule of adult (post-involutional) hosts, it was observed that graft growth actually exceeded the growth rate of the thymus in normal C57Bl mice from the age of 1 day to 4 weeks (METCALF, WAKONIG-VAARTAJA and BRADLEY, 1964). This is strongly suggestive that if systemic inhibitory influences do increase in post-involutional life, their effect on thymic lymphoid proliferation must be minimal.

Perhaps the strongest evidence against systemic influences being responsible for thymus involution is the fact that none of these systemic influences alter the time of onset of age involution—merely the absolute weight changes involved (DOUGHERTY, 1952).

Our present conception of the role of systemic influences on thymic lymphopoiesis is that these influences are not responsible for determining the high mitotic activity of thymic cells nor are they primarily responsible for age, strain and sex differences in thymus weight or mitotic activity. In the normal animal these general influences may slightly affect the level at which thymic lymphopoiesis is operating, but the basic proliferative drive stimulating thymic lymphopoiesis must emanate from within the thymus itself.

3. Nature of Intrinsic Thymic Factors Stimulating Lymphopoiesis

Thymus grafts have proved particularly valuable in the analysis of thymic factors responsible for stimulating thymic lymphopoiesis. All established thymus grafts are chimaeric organs—the epithelial and reticulum cell elements being donor in origin, and the lymphoid cells being derived from the host. This allows graft experiments to be designed which can indicate the influence exerted by either population in determining organ growth and cellular proliferative activity.

As was described earlier the thymus is basically an epithelial and reticulum cell "sponge" embedded in which are lymphoid cells. Thymus graft data make it clear that the carrying capacity of this thymic sponge (the size of the sponge) limits the amount of lymphoid tissue which can be present in the thymus. When one quarter or one half of a thymus is grafted, the maximum size attainable by the graft is exactly one quarter or one half of that attainable by a whole thymus graft. Similarly when more than one thymus is grafted to the same recipient, the total mass of thymus graft tissue bears a strict linear relationship with the number of organs grafted (Table 3) (METCALF, 1963). In support of this concept of the size limiting nature of the carrying capacity of the thymic sponge is the fact that partial thymectomy is not followed by regeneration of the portion remaining, which neither increases in size nor exhibits increased mitotic activity (METCALF, 1964). However when the epithelial and reticulum cell spongework of the thymus is made to collapse inwards by destroying the cortical lymphoid cells (e.g. by cortisone administration), then after repopulation, the thymus promptly regenerates to pretreatment size (ISHIDATE and METCALF, 1963).

It seems probable that isolated pieces of thymic spongework can function independently. Thus when a single thymus is minced into small fragments before grafting, each fragment can survive and increase in size (to a limit related to the initial fragment size) provided only that some medullary tissue is present in each fragment (METCALF, 1963). Fragments of cortical tissue are unable to survive as thymus tissue after grafting. The minimal size of a functional thymic sub unit is not known. It may be the thymic lobule which, as pointed out earlier, is of remarkably uniform size throughout the various species. It could however be much smaller—merely a segment of such a lobule, since this could provide both medullary tissue and cortical framework tissue. We have never been able to obtain successful thymus grafts after breaking down the donor organ into a single cell suspension, even when such a suspension was placed in a single subcutaneous pocket. However it is difficult to ensure that such grafted cell suspensions remain localised as a cell aggregate in the subcutaneous tissues and such a procedure might produce successful grafts if some improved method could be devised for keeping the cells concentrated in one locus.

What is the evidence that the epithelial and reticulum cell meshwork actually *stimulates* lymphopoiesis in the thymus cortex?

When neonatal thymus grafts were placed in very old recipient animals it was observed that graft lymphocyte mitotic indices were higher than those in the host thymus. Since both types of thymus tissue were repopulated by host cells (of the same age) and resided in the same hormonal and nutritional internal environment, the only differences involved were in the age and functional activity of the epithelial and reticulum cell elements of the two thymus tissues. Thus the young thymic framework elements must have exerted a true proliferative stimulus which was also more powerful than that exerted by the older framework cells.

Similarly when parental thymus grafts from strains AKR and C3H (in which there is a strain difference in the mitotic indices of the thymic lymphoid cells) were placed in (AKR × C3H)F_1 hosts, it was found that the AKR graft lymphoid cells had higher mitotic indices than those of the C3H grafts (METCALF, 1962). Both graft tissues were repopulated by similar F_1 lymphoid cells and both resided in the same F_1 environment. The different mitotic indices in the two types of graft must have been due to different degrees of stimulation by the surviving parental epithelial and reticulum cells in the grafts—again indicating the existence of a proliferative stimulus emanating from these tissues.

It is apparent that this proliferative stimulus emanating from the epithelial and reticulum cell meshwork is not subject to specific feedback inhibition by the body. Thymus grafts from very young donors exhibit intense mitotic activity at a time when the host thymus mitotic activity may be falling sharply due to age involution. Further, the mitotic activity exhibited by thymus graft lymphoid cells in multiple thymus grafted mice is as high as the mitotic activity in single thymus grafts even when extraordinary amounts of thymus graft tissue are present in the same animal (MATSUYAMA, WIADROWSKI and METCALF, 1966). This intense mitotic activity of the thymus grafts also has no effect on mitotic activity of the host thymus.

If a similar type of experiment is performed with spleen grafts, the results clearly indicate that the body can regulate, either by an active process or by a passive process of demand and supply, the amount of spleen tissue present in the body. Single spleen grafts attain a larger size in splenectomised than in sham operated hosts (METCALF, 1963 b) and when progressively more and more spleen grafts are placed in the same splenectomised host, the size attained by each graft becomes progressively smaller, the total mass of spleen graft tissue reaching a plateau which approximates the weight of the normal spleen (METCALF, 1964 d).

In the case of thymus grafts and thymus tissue, either no cells or humoral products are released to the body to activate a specific inhibitory feedback mechanism or no such mechanism exists to be activated. Since a humoral factor and almost certainly some lymphoid cells are released into the body from thymus tissue it seems more likely that there exists no specific target or receptor tissue in the body capable of detecting these products and producing a specific substance inhibiting the production or activity of the intrinsic stimulating factor. Since systemic inhibitory factors for thymic lymphopoiesis *are* produced in the body (e.g. adrenal corticosteroids) it is apparent that products from thymus tissue do not stimulate an increased secretion of these systemic inhibitory hormones which could then reduce thymic proliferative activity.

In this context the intrinsic stimulation of lymphopoiesis within each piece of thymus tissue operates autonomously—being independent of specific inhibition by neighbouring grafts, host thymus or other host tissues. From what has been said of the growth potential of thymus fragments it is probable that the autonomous unit of thymus tissue is much smaller than the whole organ itself—probably a sub unit of lobule which includes both medullary and cortical tissue.

During adult life potential thymic lymphoid stem cells seed out from the circulation into the interstices of the epithelial and reticulum cell spongework in the thymus cortex. The anatomical arrangement of the epithelial sheaths around the vessels is such that gaps are present in these sheaths particularly in the outer part of the cortex and this is the possible site of entry of these blood-borne immigrant cells. It is now known that other potential stem cells for the erythroid, myeloid and megakarocytic series of cells also circulate in the blood. It is uncertain whether these are distinct cell populations or whether there is but one multi-potent type of potential stem cell. However in chronic myeloid leukaemia in humans it is known that the abnormal Philadelphia chromosome occurs in the primitive myeloid and erythroid cells but not in the lymphoid cells (WHANG et al., 1963). Further, it is known that suspensions of thymic or lymph node lymphocytes are not capable of giving rise to erythroid or myeloid cells when injected into lethally irradiated recipients. This suggests that there are at least two distinct populations of circulating potential stem cells: 1. lymphoid, and 2. erythroid/myeloid.

Erythropoiesis and myelopoiesis do not occur in the normal thymus but it is not known whether or not the precursor cells for these cell lines enter the thymus. It may be that the thymus possesses a barrier allowing only the entry of lymphoid precursor cells, or alternatively all types of precursor cells may enter the thymus but only the lymphoid type cells find a suitable environment in which to proliferate and differentiate.

HARRIS and FORD (1964) observed seeding of thymus graft cells only to lymph nodes and not to bone marrow or spleen, whereas bone marrow and spleen cells, but not lymph node cells, seeded in the thymus of irradiated mice (FORD and MICKLEM, 1963). This might occur if the thymus only selects from the circulating cells specific cells capable of seeding in the thymus, but these same cells also may be capable of seeding in lymph nodes (either before or after residence in the thymus). However, there may be a separate population of lymphoid precursor cells capable only of seeding in lymph node and spleen but not in the thymus.

In view of these uncertainties it cannot be stated positively that the thymus exerts a specific *lymphopoietic* proliferative stimulus on previously uncommitted multi-potential stem cells, merely that potential lymphoid stem cells seed in the thymus and there are stimulated to proliferate and differentiate.

The anatomical concentration of lymphocyte mitotic activity in the peripheral regions of the cortex of the thymic lobule and along the radial vessels in the cortex in thymus grafts suggests either that it is in these regions that the incoming stem cells lodge, or that the epithelial cells enclosing the outer aspect of the lobule and forming the sheaths of the radial vessels are themselves involved in the stimulation of lymphocyte mitotic activity.

It was mentioned earlier that cortical lymphocyte mitotic activity also is concentrated around, and in some way dependent on cell contact with, the PAS-positive reticulum cells of the cortex. These cells survive in the thymus grafts (METCALF and ISHIDATE, 1962) and are thus able to exert their potential influence on repopulating cells in grafts, a necessary requisite for including this cell type in the epithelial and reticulum cell complex postulated to regulate thymic lymphopoiesis. The exact nature of the interaction between PAS cells and lymphocytes is unknown. The PAS cells appear to trigger off, or initiate, the mitotic event in lymphoid cells in contact with them, but they may possibly exert a true stimulus to proliferate—that is by initiating DNA synthesis in these cells. The active material in PAS cells is unknown, but the prominent PAS-positive granules may be the active principle. If this is so it is of interest that both the medullary epithelial cells and, to a lesser degree, the reticular epithelial cells secrete a superficially similar PAS-positive material. The PAS cells are known to be phagocytic and their PAS-positive granules may have been acquired by phagocytosis of PAS-positive lymphocyte stimulating material produced initially by the epithelial cells.

Reutilisation by lymphocytes of breakdown products from other lymphocytes is well known in the thymus and in other lymphoid organs and occurs to such a degree as to present technical problems when analysing tritiated thymidine labelling data. It is conceivable that the availability of these breakdown products could be a rate limiting factor in lymphopoiesis. It is a curious fact that the frequency of pyknotic lymphocytes in lymph node or spleen germinal centres parallels the degree of local mitotic activity, and in the thymus pyknotic cells are present in considerable numbers even during active thymic growth in early life (METCALF, 1964). The PAS cells are of course not the only cells in the thymus phagocytosing lymphocyte debris, nevertheless in the normal thymus at any one time about one third of these cells contain lymphocytes in the process of being broken down. In cortisone-treated mice this phagocytic activity of PAS cells becomes greatly intensified and phagocytosed lymphocytes are rapidly broken down in the cytoplasm, possibly with the formation of additional PAS granular material. When regeneration commences a few days later there is an increased amount of lymphocyte mitotic activity associated with the PAS cells (ISHIDATE and METCALF, 1963). It is possible therefore that at least part of the association of PAS cells and lymphocyte mitotic activity may come from the fact that the PAS cells are making lymphocyte breakdown products available to other dividing lymphoid cells. This would constitute a type of direct feedback regulation of lymphopoiesis by lymphocyte breakdown products—the greater the cell destruction, the greater the stimulation of lymphopoiesis.

The PAS cells are scattered at fairly regular intervals throughout the outer part of the cortex in a ratio of approximately one PAS cell to every two hundred lymphocytes. This group of cells—a PAS cell with its attendant lymphocytes—may constitute some type of functional unit but it is more likely, in view of the failure of cortical fragments alone to survive grafting, that the autonomous proliferative sub units of thymic tissue are larger and include some medullary tissue.

Since medullary epithelial cells have been shown to be necessary for thymus tissue growth and since an association has been described between the cortical reticular epithelial cells and lymphocyte mitotic activity, it is surprising that lymphocyte mitotic activity in the medulla is minimal. This would suggest that if epithelial cells do produce a proliferative stimulus, it cannot stimulate lymphoid cells unless they are residing in a suitable environment—specifically in the cortex rather than in the medulla.

However an alternative explanation is possible for the low medullary lymphocyte mitotic activity—namely that the medullary lymphoid cells are a distinct population, not related to the cortical lymphoid cells. It is claimed by LEBLOND and SAINTE MARIE (1960) that cortical cells migrate through the medulla, which would imply that cortical and medullary lymphocytes were members of the same cell population. However it has been shown that the medullary lymphoid cells are much more radioresistant than cortical cells (TROWELL, 1961) and a similar resistance of medullary lymphocytes has been observed to the lymphocytolytic effects of cortisone (ISHIDATE and METCALF, 1963). It is possible that many of the medullary lymphoid cells may be lymph node type lymphocytes in free exchange with the recirculating lymphocytes of the body. Certainly in mice with generalised reticulum cell sarcoma, the medullary lymphoid tissue of the thymus can be infiltrated by sarcoma cells along with the lymph nodes and spleen but the thymus cortex is rarely involved. In graft versus host disease following the injection of foreign lymphoid cells, the proliferating groups of large pyroninophilic cells seen in this disease in the spleen and lymph nodes may often also be observed in the thymus medulla but again not in the thymus cortex. Similarly in autoradiographic studies on thymic lymphopoiesis, some evidence was obtained for the existence of a small population of small lymphocytes in the thymus having a longer life span than the majority of the small lymphocytes. From the appearance of autoradiographs of sections of these thymus glands, it seemed evident that this secondary population of long lived small lymphocytes was located in the medulla (MATSUYAMA, WIADROWSKI and METCALF, 1966). If the medullary lymphocytes represent a distinct population from the cortical lymphocytes, they may also differ in that the medullary lymphocytes are insusceptible to stimulation by the intrinsic thymic proliferative stimulus.

Finally, as was discussed earlier, CLARK (1965) has recently produced evidence suggesting functional differences between cortical and medullary epithelial cells, and these differences may be connected with the question of whether or not the cells produce lymphocyte mitotic stimulating material.

So far in this discussion of the regulation of thymic lymphopoiesis we have discussed the regulation of thymus size and of thymic mitotic activity and have seen that these two parameters of the thymus are not necessarily related, although they may be regulated by the same epithelial-reticulum cell complex. There remains a third aspect of thymic lymphopoiesis warranting discussion—the regulation of differentiation in the proliferating lymphoid cells.

In the adult thymus the proportions of large to medium to small lymphocytes are fixed and quite characteristic. Under what conditions is the pattern varied and what mechanisms determine this pattern of differentiation?

In the young, actively growing thymus, the proportions of primitive large and medium cells are far higher than in adult life. Thus in one day old AKR thymuses there are approximately 3% large lymphocytes and 30—40% medium lymphocytes versus 1% and 10% of these respective cells in the adult thymus. This implies that in the very young thymus, more daughter cells of primitive cells tend to remain primitive than in adult life, providing the basis for the expanding population size of the thymus as it grows in early life. A similar situation is seen during regeneration of the adult thymus. Initially the proportions of large and medium to small lymphocytes are higher than normal but as the weight of the regenerating thymus approaches normal again, the proportions of primitive lymphoid cells fall back to the normal adult values (ISHIDATE and METCALF, 1963).

Obviously some mechanism exists in the thymus for regulating the ratio of daughter type to parental type offspring and this mechanism is capable of flexibility when meeting the demands of growth and regeneration. At the cellular level it seems that most cells when dividing tend to produce daughter cells which are similar rather than dissimilar (LEBLOND, 1964). Thus a large lymphocyte would probably produce either two large lymphocyte daughter cells or two medium lymphocyte daughter cells rather than that each large lymphocyte produces one large and one medium daughter lymphocyte.

As with the regulation of mitotic activity, it is probable that the regulation of differentiation is enforced by the epithelial and reticulum cells of the thymus, but the mechanisms employed are unknown. Cell contact processes seem unlikely in view of the motile nature of the lymphocyte, and differentiation may be regulated humorally by a type of biological mass action similar to chemical mass action. At a certain level of differentiating factor produced by the epithelial and reticulum cell complex a certain probability may exist that say 50% of dividing large lymphocytes will form medium lymphocytes and if the level of the differentiating factor rises then this probability may rise to say 70%. It is conceivable that a single differentiating factor could regulate both large and medium lymphocytes. This system would envisage the effect as being entirely random throughout the proliferating cell population rather than that foci of large lymphocytes in one region give rise only to large lymphocyte offspring and that other foci give rise only to medium lymphocyte offspring. Certainly there is no histological evidence to support such a concept of local areas of specialised cell division.

Logically this process of differentiation should be subject to some feedback regulation, to maintain constant proportions of large to medium to small cells. Thus medium and small lymphocytes may produce some metabolite which operates to cut down the effective level of differentiating factor, either by cutting down the production of the factor or perhaps neutralising it, or alternatively the medium and small lymphocytes may actually metabolise the factor, reducing its concentration in the cortex.

If there is a differentiation feedback mechanism it must operate on a purely local level, since the presence of thymus graft tissue in an animal has no influence on differentiation on the host thymus or in other thymus graft tissue.

This process of regulation of cellular differentiation is probably also influenced by circulating hormones and it is likely for example that the adrenal corticosteroids could be involved, if only as a supplementary influence on a local thymic regulatory process.

Our understanding of the exact mechanisms involved in the differentiation of dividing lymphoid cells will probably remain rudimentary until satisfactory methods are devised for maintaining thymic lymphocytes and fragments of thymus in tissue culture where some of these possibilities can be examined experimentally.

Our present conception of the regulation of lymphopoiesis in the thymus is shown diagrammatically in Fig. 21. Lymphoid precursor cells enter the thymus from the blood and there come under a proliferative stimulus exerted by the combined interaction of at least three cell types—the medullary epithelial cells, the cortical reticular epithelial cells and the PAS cells. This same cell complex also appears to regulate differentiation in the dividing lymphoid cells. The situation in the thymus may well be an analogue of that operating in the regulation of erythropoiesis. In erythropoiesis, a humoral factor erythropoietin is produced (mainly by the kidney) which circulates in the blood and can induce potential erythropoietic stem cells to commence haemo-

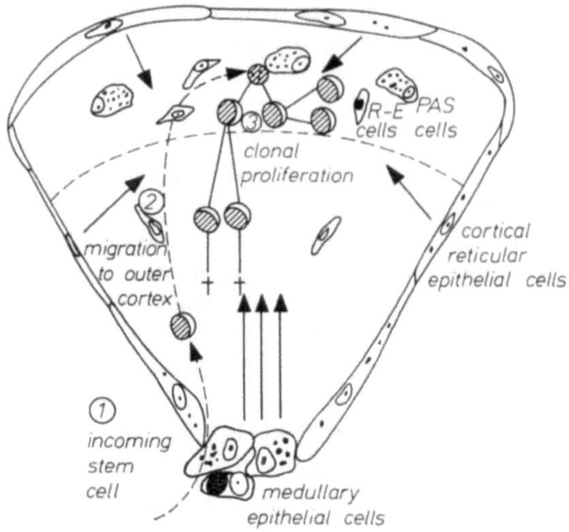

Fig. 21. Schematic representation of factors regulating lymphopoiesis in the thymus cortex. New stem cells enter the cortex from the blood and in the outer part of the cortex come under the influence of an intrinsic proliferative stimulus, probably of medullary epithelial cell origin. The microenvironment in the cortex allowing responsiveness to this stimulation and probably regulating differentiation is conditioned by the cortical reticular epithelial cells and reticuloendothelial cells including the PAS cells

globin synthesis and cell division to form mature red cells. This action of erythropoietin on erythroid stem cells only occurs when the stem cells are located in a microenvironment which allows them to respond to stimulation (e.g. in the bone marrow or the mouse spleen). The special nature of the microenvironment in these locations is probably determined by a stromal cell complex which subsequently may also regulate differentiation in the dividing cells. In the thymus, the epithelial cells may produce a humoral factor "lymphopoietin" which can stimulate division of potential lymphoid stem cells provided they are located in the interstices of the cortical meshwork. The reticular epithelial cells and reticulum cells of this meshwork might not only condition the microenvironment to allow the lymphoid cells to respond by proliferation but might also subsequently regulate the degree of differentiation occurring in these dividing cells. This intrinsic thymic regulatory system is autonomous and appears not to be subject to specific feedback inhibition by the body. Fluctuations in the strength and nature of the intrinsic proliferative stimulus appear to be responsible for the age changes occurring in thymus size and mitotic activity.

Summary

Thymus size and mitotic activity can be influenced by the supply of thymus-repopulating cells and by general hormonal and nutritional influences. However these factors appear to be of secondary importance only. Thymic lymphopoiesis is stimulated primarily by an intrinsic stimulus emanating from the epithelial-reticulum cell complex in the thymus which also may regulate lymphocyte differentiation. The size (carrying capacity) of this cell complex limits the number of lymphoid cells contained in the thymus. The intrinsic thymic proliferative stimulus is not subject to feedback regulation but the strength of the stimulus varies with the age, strain and sex of the animal.

Chapter 5

Effect of the Thymus on Peripheral Lymphoid Organs

The term "peripheral lymphoid organs" needs some explanation. As has been described earlier, there is a distinct dichotomy in the response of the different lymphoid organs to antigenic stimulation—the lymph nodes, splenic lymphoid follicles and the Peyer's patches responding by hyperplasia and increased mitotic activity, but the thymus exhibiting no morphological changes. The blood lymphocytes seem also to be part of the antigen-responsive group of lymphoid organs since their number is influenced by antigenic stimulation and the work of GOWANS has clearly shown that (excluding the thymus) lymphocytes recirculate from one lymphoid organ to another via the blood (GOWANS and KNIGHT, 1964). It has also been mentioned that many workers feel that the thymus is a central factory producing lymphocytes which are distributed to lymphoid organs around the body.

The term "peripheral lymphoid organs" is used as a useful phrase to cover those lymphoid organs scattered around the body which differ from the thymus in being responsive to antigenic stimulation and which may also be the recipients of cells exported from the centrally located thymus.

Does the thymus exert any influence on the size or functional activity of these peripheral lymphoid organs? Theoretically several methods could be used to investigate this question—1. to observe the effects of thymectomy, 2. to observe the effects of thymus grafts and 3. to observe the effects of thymus extracts. All three approaches have been used by various investigators and the results of these studies will now be reviewed.

1. Effect of Thymectomy

Historically, one of the first experiments on thymus function was carried out by PATON and GOODALL (1904). These workers studied the effect on the lymphoid tissues of thymectomy in neonatal guinea pigs—animals which were suitable for such a study, because the thymus occupies a subcutaneous cervical location in the guinea pig. They obtained evidence that blood lymphocyte levels decreased to 30% following thymectomy. Somewhat conflicting data were produced later by GYLLENSTEN (1953) who reported that subtotal thymectomy in guinea pigs resulted in a slight hyperplasia of the lymphoid organs. Subsequent to these early investigations, there has been a remarkable degree of unanimity in observations made on the effects of thymectomy in various species.

METCALF (1959 a, 1960) reported that thymectomy in four weeks old C57Bl mice was followed by the slow development during the following eight weeks of a moderate degree of lymphopenia (lymphocyte levels falling to 30—50% below control levels) (Fig. 22) and a corresponding degree of weight loss in the spleen and subcutaneous lymph nodes. These changes did not develop immediately after thymec-

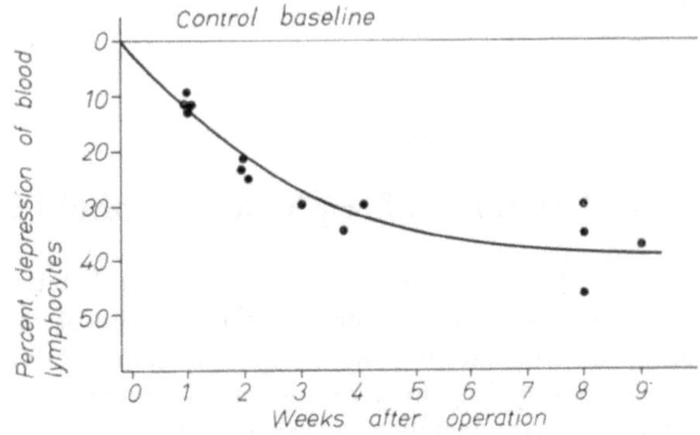

Fig. 22. Lymphopenia developing in C57Bl mice following thymectomy at the age of five weeks. Each point represents mean value of four experimental mice compared with four control mice

tomy but slowly reached a maximum two to three months after operation, at which time the lymphoid organs appeared to reach a new state of equilibrium. Histological examination of the lymph nodes and spleen lymphoid follicles from such thymectomised mice revealed that not all cell components were equally affected in the post-thymectomy atrophy. For example, in the spleen there was no diminution in the total number of lymphoid follicles or in their average size. Germinal centres were equally frequent in the lymphoid follicles of thymectomised and sham operated mice, but the mitotic activity of the primitive cells of the germinal centres was reduced in thymectomised animals to about 50% of that in control germinal centres (Table 4). The

Table 4. *Effect of Thymectomy at 4 Weeks of Age on C 57 Bl Spleen Lymphoid Tissue* [1]

Operation	No. of mice	Mean spleen weight mgm	Mean % spleen occupied by lymphoid tissue	Mean % follicles with germinal centres	Mean No. mitoses per germinal centre	Central follicle area	
						Mean No. lymphoid cells per field	Mean % small lymphocytes in field
Sham thymectomy	15	101 ± 19 [2]	26 ± 5	53 ± 9	2.6 ± 0.5	40 ± 6	92%
Thymectomy	13	75 ± 18	26 ± 7	53 ± 17	1.7 ± 0.6	28 ± 5	78%
Statistical significance of difference		P<0.01	N.S.	N.S.	P<0.01	P<0.01	P<0.01

[1] Mice examined three months after thymectomy.
[2] ± Standard deviation.

most characteristic feature however was a reduction in the number of small lymphocytes in the lymphoid follicles, particularly in the region of the central arteriole of the follicle (Figs. 23 and 24). In some cases the small lymphocyte depletion was so severe as to cause a "motheaten" appearance in the central region of the follicle.

The population of primitive lymphocytes did not appear to be depleted by thymectomy. Similar changes were observed in lymph node architecture, and again the most obvious changes were a depletion of small lymphocytes in the dense lymphoid aggre-

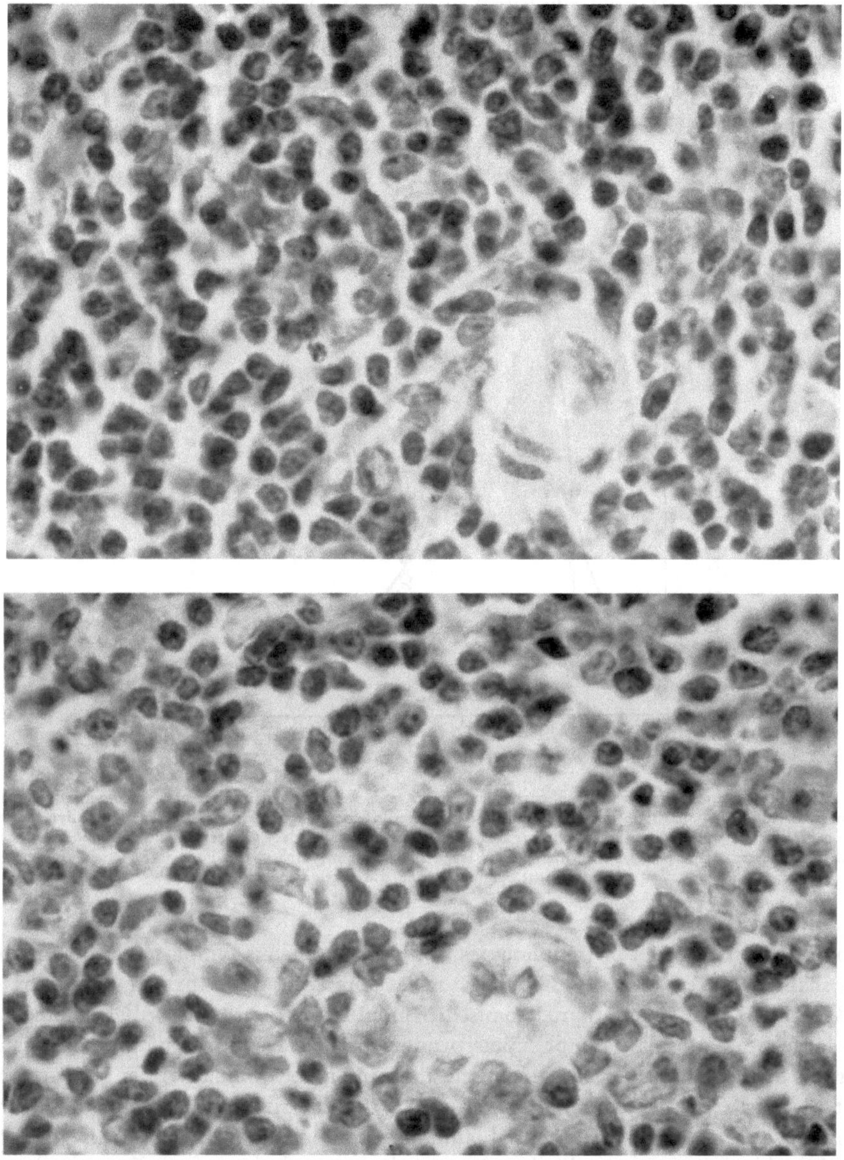

Fig. 23/24. High power view of central arteriolar region of spleen lymphoid follicle in a sham thymectomised (upper) and in a thymectomised (lower) C57Bl mouse, three months after operation. Note depletion of small lymphocytes and relative increase in large and medium lymphocytes in thymectomised animal. H and E ×1200 (reduced to $^9/_{10}$)

gates in the cortical regions of the lymph node and a reduction in mitotic activity of the lymph node germinal centres. Plasma cells and reticulum cells were not decreased in numbers in these tissues and may possibly even have been increased in number although the overall reduction in the size of the organs made this difficult to assess.

These findings on the effect of adult thymectomy on the spleen and lymph nodes in mice have recently been confirmed in detail by NAKAKUKI and NISHIZUKA (1964) working with AKR strain mice.

Recently we have reinvestigated the effect of adult thymectomy in the mouse on the population of lymphocytes in the subcutaneous and mesenteric lymph nodes and the spleen by preparing cell suspensions from such organs and examining them with a Model B Coulter counter (METCALF, unpublished data). In Fig. 25 is shown the

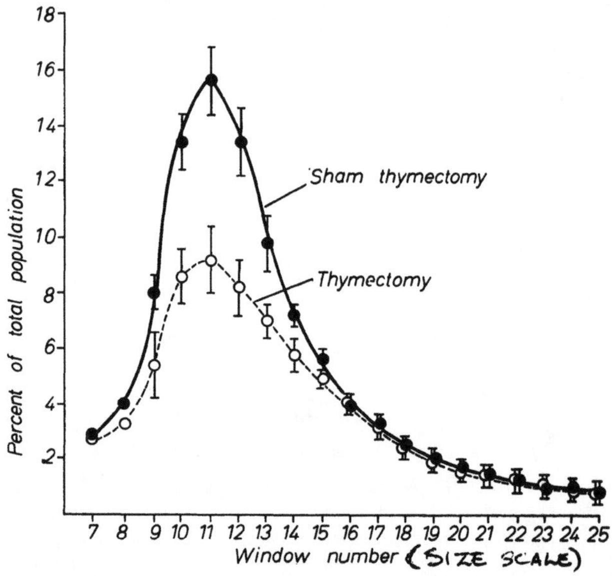

Fig. 25. Coulter counter analysis of subcutaneous lymph node cell populations from thymectomised and sham thymectomised (AKR×C57Bl)F_1 mice five months after operation at the age of six weeks. Data from thymectomised mice corrected for weight decrease of the organs. Note that there is a selective decrease in the population size of small lymphocytes (large peak) but no increase in large and medium lymphocytes. Each point is mean value of six mice, vertical bars are standard deviations of values

population distribution of lymphocytes in the subcutaneous lymph nodes of 6 months old sham operated (AKR × C57Bl)F_1 mice compared with that in 6 months old (AKR × C57Bl)F_1 mice, thymectomised 5 months previously. It will be noted that the large peak of small lymphocytes prominent in the control lymph nodes is less marked in the cell suspensions from the thymectomised animals. It is also apparent that there is a greater degree of heterogeneity in the size of the lymph node small lymphocytes in the thymectomised animals than in the controls. It is uncertain whether this represents a selective decrease in a population of medium sized small lymphocytes or an overall increase in the heterogeneity of the size of all small lymphocytes. When these data from the thymectomised mice were corrected for the smaller size of the thymectomised lymph nodes, it was evident that the total number of large and medium cells in the lymph nodes of thymectomised mice was normal whilst the total number of small lymphocytes was selectively reduced. A similar depletion of small lymphocytes and an increase in heterogeneity of surviving small lymphocytes was also observed in the mesenteric lymph node and the spleen of thymectomised mice.

NAKAMOTO (1957) reported that thymectomy in young adult rabbits was followed by the development of a lymphopenia and a decrease in the lymphocytes in the efferent lymph from the popliteal lymph nodes. He also noted atrophy of lymph nodes in such animals. REINHARDT and YOFFEY (1956) reported that 40 days after thymectomy in adult guinea pigs, the thoracic duct output of lymphocytes had fallen from 18.86×10^6 per hour to 8.44×10^6 per hour. BIERRING (1960) also reported that adult thymectomy in rats led to a fall in thoracic duct output but not to a measurable fall in lymph node weights or mitotic activity.

SCHOOLEY and KELLY (1964) demonstrated that thymectomy at 6 days of age in rats had reduced thoracic duct lymphocyte output to 27% and had caused lymph node weight loss and lymphopenia, when the rats were examined two months later. Thymectomy at 4 weeks of age also led to a reduced thoracic duct lymphocyte output but to no lymph node weight loss. Evidence was presented by SCHOOLEY and KELLY that thymic lymphocytes probably do not enter the thoracic duct lymph directly from the thymus and that the reduced thoracic duct output of lymphocytes following thymectomy is probably a secondary effect following on an overall reduction in lymphoid organ mass and lymphocyte recirculation.

Little attention seems to have been paid to the effect of adult thymectomy on bone marrow lymphocytes, however BIERRING (1963) observed that adult thymectomy in rats had no effect on bone marrow lymphocytes nor did thymectomy combined with partial lymph node resection. BIERRING also observed that mitotic activity was not increased in the lymph nodes left *in situ* after the latter type of combined operation.

Studies have also been made on the effect of adult thymectomy in mice combined with whole body irradiation. MILLER, DOAK and CROSS (1963) reported that adult thymectomy was followed by the development of lymphopenia and that the degree of lymphopenia was accentuated by whole body irradiation. Bone marrow injections did not improve the lymphopenic state but did allow survival of the mice when the dose of irradiation used was lethal (850 r) by providing erythropoietic and myelopoietic cells for the animals.

GLOBERSON and FELDMANN (1964) reported that 550 r whole body irradiation led to lymphoid organ atrophy followed by regeneration of the lymphoid tissues. Thymectomy combined with 550 r whole body irradiation reduced the number of lymphoid follicles in the regenerating spleen and those which did reappear exhibited reduced cellularity and mitotic activity. By contrast, erythropoiesis and myelopoiesis appeared more extensive in the regenerating spleens in thymectomised irradiated mice than in those subjected to irradiation alone. In some spleens from thymectomised irradiated mice, confluent sheets or nodules of erythropoietic tissue were observed, an appearance never seen in control irradiated mice. Erythropoiesis appeared earlier and regression of these elements was more retarded in thymectomised irradiated mice than in control irradiated mice. Thymus grafts placed in thymectomised irradiated mice restored a normal lymphoid regeneration pattern. In a similar study AUERBACH (1963) demonstrated that thymectomy combined with 900 r irradiation in (C3H $\times$ AKR)F_1 mice prevented the regeneration of spleen lymphoid follicles.

MILLER in 1961 while observing the effects of thymectomy in neonatal (less than 1 day old) mice on lymphoid leukaemia development noted that thymectomy at this age produced dramatic changes in blood lymphocyte levels and lymph node and spleen morphology (MILLER, 1961; 1962). Simultaneously ARCHER and PIERCE (1961), ARCHER et al. (1962) and GOOD et al. (1962) working on the effect of thymectomy on immune responses also performed thymectomies on newborn rabbits and mice and, apart from observing changes in immunological responsiveness in such animals which will be discussed later, observed similar changes in the lymphoid tissues to those noted by MILLER. Subsequently WAKSMAN, ARNASON and JANKOVIC (1962) made a detailed study in rats of the effects of neonatal thymectomy on the lymphoid organs. The changes described by this group have now been confirmed repeatedly by others in rats and mice and also by studies in hamsters, and a reasonably clear picture of the effects of neonatal thymectomy in various species has now emerged.

Following neonatal thymectomy in mice, as after thymectomy in adult life, little change is observed in the lymphoid organs for several weeks. These organs increase in size at a normal rate and contain dense follicular aggregates of small lymphocytes and active germinal centres. However, blood lymphocyte levels do show an immediate response to thymectomy. In newborn mice, lymphocyte levels in the blood are relatively low and normally increase rapidly in the first ten days of life. In neonatally thymectomised mice, lymphocyte levels tend to remain at the initial low levels, showing little increase with increasing age of the animal. MILLER (1964 a) reported that the small lymphocytes of the blood are more severely affected by neonatal thymectomy than the large lymphocytes, whilst polymorph and monocyte levels remain normal. After several weeks (the length of the latent period varying from one strain of mouse to another, and from one species to another) the lymphoid organs of neonatally thymectomised animals begin to lose weight. Histologically these atrophic lymphoid organs contain reduced numbers of lymphoid follicles and germinal centres but, as with adult thymectomy, the most dramatic change is seen in the small lymphocyte population. The central areas of the spleen lymphoid follicles are severely depleted of small lymphocytes and in the lymph nodes there is a marked reduction in the small lymphocyte population in the normally densely populated outer cortical region of the lymph node. Plasma cell and reticulum cell populations in the lymph nodes are not reduced by thymectomy and in many studies some evidence for an actual increase in the numbers of these cells has been obtained. The non-lymphoid elements in the spleen—the erythroid, myeloid, megakaryocytic and reticulum cells—do not appear to be affected consistently by neonatal thymectomy. In some thymectomised animals an overall reduction in the number of these cells has been observed but in others a probable increase in these cells occurred. This variability in the response of these non lymphoid tissues is almost certainly an indirect secondary effect of thymectomy and is related to the decline in health of animals following neonatal thymectomy, a question which we shall return to later.

Thus the changes in lymphoid organs caused by adult and neonatal thymectomy are essentially similar qualitatively, the difference being that neonatal thymectomy leads to a more rapid development of lymphoid organ atrophy and to a more severe degree of depletion of lymphocytes in these organs than does adult thymectomy.

MILLER and HOWARD (1964) reported that neonatal thymectomy in their strains of mice was followed by hyperplasia of the reticuloendothelial system, and reticulum cells and histiocytes were present in increased numbers in the lymph node, spleen and liver. Splenomegaly was often observed and was due in part to increased extra-medullary haemopoiesis. The phagocytic index of reticulo-endothelial tissues as assessed by carbon clearance was also found to be higher in neonatally thymectomised than in control mice. It is uncertain how many of these finding are the direct result of thymectomy and how many are due to ill health and infections which occur following neonatal thymectomy.

Because of technical difficulties, thymectomy in mice and rats has rarely been performed later than the first two or three months of life. It is not known therefore whether or not thymectomy performed in middle age or old age is followed by demonstrable changes in the peripheral lymphoid organs.

Recently a study has been made of blood lymphocytes following thymectomy in humans with myasthenia gravis (Joske, 1958; Dameshek, 1965). In these patients thymectomy was followed by the development of a moderate degree of lymphopenia.

Two features of the effect of thymectomy on the peripheral lymphoid organs need emphasis. In the immediate post-operative period, even after neonatal thymectomy, there is *no* observable effect on the lymphoid organs. If the thymus simply functions as a factory producing about half the small lymphocytes of the body (as is indicated by direct mitotic counts), and if these cells have free access to peripheral lymphoid organs, then thymectomy should be followed rapidly by detectable falls in the levels of small lymphocytes in other organs. The only mechanism which could compensate for the loss of half the body's production of small lymphocytes following thymectomy and prevent the immediate development of a lymphopenic state, would be the ability of non-thymic small lymphocytes in a thymectomised animal to increase their life span to twice that of lymphocytes in a normal animal. However, autoradiographic data obtained in our laboratory from C57Bl mice, thymectomised in adult life, have given no indication of an increased small lymphocyte life span in the blood or lymph nodes (Metcalf and Matsuyama, unpublished data). In fact, as has been discussed earlier, the evidence is now against a simple "factory" concept of thymus function and suggests that very few cells produced in the thymus ever leave this organ. If this is so, it is much easier to explain the fact that there is no *immediate* change in the lymphoid organs following thymectomy.

The second noteworthy feature of the effects of thymectomy is the fact that when a lymphopenic state does develop, the degree of lymphopenia does not continue to increase progressively with time. At least following adult thymectomy, after the development of a certain degree of lymphocyte depletion in the lymphoid organs, these organs reach a new level of equilibrium after which the lymphocyte content of the various organs remains relatively constant. In the case of neonatally thymectomised animals, lymphocyte depletion appears to be progressive but the interpretation of these changes is complicated by the fact that animals subsequently become sick and in such animals the progressive nature of the lymphopenia is almost certainly the secondary result of the onset of fatal illness in these animals. It seems reasonable to conclude that the non-thymic lymphoid tissues of an animal are capable of a certain level of functional and proliferative activity in the absence of a thymic influence—whether this be cell export or non-cellular influence. This fact needs to be remembered when the immunological effects of thymectomy are considered.

Whilst the effects of adult thymectomy in causing lymphoid organ atrophy do not appear to be progressive, it is equally true that no subsequent regeneration of these atrophic organs occurs with the passage of time. We have studied recently the lymphoid organs in old mice (aged 18—24 months) which were thymectomised at the age of six weeks, and have observed the persistence of relative lymphoid atrophy and small lymphocyte depletion in these organs of the same magnitude as was observed at earlier time intervals after thymectomy.

Thymectomy appears to be an ideal method for investigating the influence of the thymus on peripheral lymphoid cell activity. Although neonatal thymectomy produces a more rapidly developing, and more severe, lymphocyte depletion than adult thymectomy, the interpretation of many of the effects of neonatal thymectomy is complicated by the development of ill health in the animals. This comment is particularly pertinent when the cell under study is the small lymphocyte which is exquisitely sensitive to the effects of infections and stress. For this reason it may be preferable in future studies on the effects of thymectomy *on small lymphocytes* to restrict observations to animals thymectomised in adult life.

2. Effect of Thymus Grafts

The state of the host lymphoid organs in mice carrying thymus grafts has been investigated in some detail in our laboratory. In adult mice examined one or two months after being grafted subcutaneously with a single isologous neonatal thymus, no changes were observed in blood lymphocyte levels or in the weights of the host thymus, spleen and mesenteric nodes (Metcalf et al., 1961). The lymph nodes draining the graft site were usually slightly heavier than the contralateral nodes but the weight differences were only 10—15%. Cytological examination of the host lymphoid organs showed no change from normal levels in thymus mitotic indices nor was any change observed in the percentage of primitive lymphoid cells or the mitotic activity of these cells in the draining lymph nodes as compared with contralateral lymph nodes (Table 5). Histologically, some draining lymph nodes showed slight

Table 5. *Effect of Subcutaneous AKR Thymus Grafts on the Weight and Cytology of (AKR×C3H)F_1 Host Subcutaneous Lymph Nodes*[1]

Organ	Mean weight mgm	Mean percentage			Combined mitotic indices of large and medium lymphocytes
		Large lymphocytes	Medium lymphocytes	Small lymphocytes	
Draining axillary lymph nodes	16±3	1.1±0.6	6.8±0.4	91.4±2.0	0.8±0.1
Contralateral axillary lymph nodes	14±2	0.6±0.2	5.4±1.1	93.6±1.0	0.7±0.2

[1] Eight mice were examined one month after grafting: Thymus grafts averaged 28 mg. in weight and were located in the left axillary region adjacent to the axillary lymph nodes.

evidence of an increased content of small lymphocytes, particularly in the peripheral and medullary sinuses, but this cell increase was minor in degree.

In animals grafted one month previously with up to 48 thymus grafts (and containing up to 1250 mg. of subcutaneous thymus graft tissue versus a total host lymphoid organ mass of approximately 250 mgm) only minor changes were observed in host lymphoid organs. There was a slight lymphocytosis in the blood (levels up to 20% higher than in control mice) and a slight (approximately 15—20%) increase in subcutaneous lymph node weights. Host thymus weights were unchanged. No correlation was observed between the mass of thymus graft tissue present and the absolute weights of host lymphoid organs (METCALF, 1963; MATSUYAMA, WIADROWSKI and METCALF, 1966). Autoradiographic studies using tritiated thymidine in 3 months old C57Bl mice carrying up to 48 neonatal thymus grafts, have shown that the presence of multiple thymus grafts in a mouse does not affect the percentage of primitive cells or the proliferative patterns of these cells in the host thymus and lymph nodes (Table 6) (MATSUYAMA, WIADROWSKI and METCALF, 1966).

Table 6. *Effect of Multiple Subcutaneous Thymus Grafts in Three Months Old C57Bl Mice on Weight, Cytology and Uptake of Tritiated Thymidine by Host Lymphoid Organs* [1]

Organ	Type of mouse	Mean organ weight mgm	Mean percent cell distribution			Mean percent cells taking up tritiated thymidine			
			Large	Medium	Small	Total cells	Large	Medium	Small
Host thymus	Control	54	1.5	7.9	90.6	11.5	87.8	69.4	0.9
	Thymus grafted	50	1.4	8.3	90.3	10.7	86.7	71.6	1.1
Thymus graft	Thymus grafted	268	1.5	8.3	90.2	10.6	86.3	71.4	1.1
Mesenteric L. N.	Control	44	0.8	3.3	95.9	3.0	79.1	54.1	0.4
	Thymus grafted	53	0.9	3.9	95.3	3.4	80.3	42.4	0.3
Subcutaneous L. N.	Control	46	0.4	2.9	96.8	1.9	80.8	39.6	0.1
	Thymus grafted	53	0.6	3.1	96.3	1.9	79.6	32.7	0.3
Blood lymphocytes	Control	—	—	—	—	0.3	—	—	0.3
	Thymus grafted	—	—	—	—	0.2	—	—	0.2

[1] Each animal grafted one month previously with 12 one day old C57Bl thymus glands. Four mice in each group. Dose of tritiated thymidine 5 uCi/gm intravenously, mice examined one hour later.

In mice carrying single thymus grafts in the subcapsular region of the kidney, no changes in host lymphoid organs were observed (METCALF, WAKONIG-VAARTAJA and BRADLEY, 1965). Mice have also been studied in which a thymus graft had been placed within the host spleen. Some of these mice developed slight splenomegaly with an increase in spleen lymphoid follicle size and germinal centre mitotic activity, but other spleens carrying thymus grafts of equal size showed no changes from normal (METCALF and BRADLEY, unpublished data).

The effects of thymectomy and thymus grafts have also been studied on the growth of spleen graft tissue in the same host. In an analysis of the effects of thymectomy on spleen graft growth, use was made of the kidney subcapsular site for spleen grafting to ensure more uniform spleen graft growth. Six weeks old C57Bl mice were thymectomised or sham operated, and one month later these mice were grafted under the kidney capsule with a single whole spleen from day old C57Bl mice. The grafted animals were killed and examined one month later. It will be seen from Table 7 that spleen graft growth was identical in thymectomised and sham

Table 7. *Growth of C57Bl Spleen Grafts Alone or Mixed with other Tissues in Various Types of Host Animal*[1]

Type of graft	Host strain	Type of host	Site of grafting	No. of animals grafted	Total spleen graft weight mg
Whole organ	C57Bl	Thymectomised one month before	Kidney subcapsular	11	47±11
Whole organ	C57Bl	Sham thymectomised one month before	Kidney subcapsular	13	48±16
Whole organ	C57Bl	Normal	Subcutaneous	10	127±50[2]
Whole organ	C57Bl	Host carrying 12 thymus grafts on other side of body.	Subcutaneous	10	111±39[2]
Minced fragments	(AKR×C57Bl)F_1	Normal	Subcutaneous	28	109±33[3]
Minced fragments mixed with thymus fragments	(AKR×C57Bl)F_1	Normal	Subcutaneous	23	182±41[3]
Minced fragments mixed with kidney fragments	(AKR×C57Bl)F_1	Normal	Subcutaneous	21	115±47[3]
Minced fragments mixed with lung fragments	(AKR×C57Bl)F_1	Normal	Subcutaneous	20	140±30[3]

[1] Spleen graft weights determined four weeks after grafting. Weight of donor neonatal spleen = 3 mgm.

[2] Total weight of 12 spleen grafts in each recipient.

[3] Total weight of 8 spleen grafts in each recipient.

operated recipients. Furthermore the size and mitotic activity of the spleen graft lymphoid follicles were also identical in the two types of host. These findings suggest strongly that in an adult host, the presence of thymus tissue does not affect the growth of neonatal spleen graft tissue, and this conclusion is strengthened by the observation that spleen graft growth, in mice grafted simultaneously with thymus grafts and spleen grafts, is not greater than in normal recipients. In these experiments, two months old C57Bl mice were grafted subcutaneously on one side of the body with 12 one day old C57Bl thymus glands and on the other side with 12 one day old C57Bl spleens. Control mice were grafted subcutaneously with 12 one day old C57Bl spleens or 12 one day old C57Bl thymus glands. The data (Table 7) indicated that spleen graft growth was identical in the two groups of mice when examined one month later.

However another type of thymus and spleen graft experiment has suggested some type of interaction between thymus and spleen graft tissue. As mentioned earlier thymus and spleen tissue can be minced and the mixture of thymus and spleen fragments when grafted together grow well, forming a graft which is a mosaic of thymus and spleen tissue. In the standard graft experiment used, eight one day old C57Bl thymus glands were minced with eight one day old C57Bl spleens and the mixture of fragments grafted subcutaneously to two months old C57Bl or (AKR × C57Bl)F_1 recipients. When these grafts were analysed one month later it was found that the thymus components of the mixed grafts had attained the same size as thymus fragments had achieved when grafted alone. However the spleen fragments in mixed grafts consistently attained a 75% larger size than when grafted alone (Table 7). This increased size seemed to affect all elements of the spleen—red pulp and lymphoid follicles alike. There was no obvious evidence of lymphocyte export from the thymus tissue to adjacent areas of spleen tissue and in fact the two tissues were usually separated either by fibrous septae or by an intact layer of thymic reticular epithelial cells. This potentiating effect of thymus graft tissue on spleen graft growth in mixed grafts was reasonably specific and a similar increased growth of spleen tissue was not seen in mixed grafts of liver or kidney tissue with spleen tissue. With mixed grafts of lung and spleen tissue, a slight increase in spleen graft growth was observed. Lung tissue grafts are characterised by the massive vascularisation they elicit from the host tissues and the improved blood supply to the mixed grafts may have been responsible for the better spleen graft growth because thymus tissue grafts also attained a slightly larger size when mixed with lung fragments than when grafted alone.

A somewhat similar finding was reported by Auerbach (1963 a) who found that culture *in vitro* of embryonic spleen fragments did not result in lymphoid follicle development, but when thymus tissue was present, increased spleen growth occurred. However Auerbach also reported a synergistic effect of the spleen fragments on thymus fragment growth and lymphoid development. This latter finding of a synergistic effect of spleen on thymus tissue was not observed by us in mixed grafts of neonatal thymus and spleen tissue. Furthermore, in many studies we have failed to demonstrate any effect of adult splenectomy or of multiple spleen grafting on thymus weight, lymphocyte differentiation or mitotic activity. It seems most unlikely, at least in the adult, that the spleen exerts any significant influence on the thymus itself.

Although host thymectomy and contralateral thymus grafting seem without influence on spleen graft growth, the mixed graft experiments and those of Auerbach suggest that thymus tissue may, under some circumstances, affect spleen graft growth. In mixed grafts, the thymus may exert some short range humoral influence on spleen cells favouring their proliferation or thymus tissue may export cells to adjacent spleen tissue, even if this is not obvious histologically. Alternatively the presence of thymus tissue adjacent to spleen tissue may allow better vascularisation of spleen graft tissue with a subsequent non specific improvement in growth—although this seems unlikely as thymus graft tissue is notably avascular, and thymus graft growth was unaffected in such mixed grafts.

3. Effect of Thymus Extracts

The third type of approach to the analysis of interactions between the thymus and peripheral lymphoid organs is to analyse the effect of thymus extracts on the lymphoid tissues. Most work along these lines has been carried out in the mouse and although the results obtained have been promising this general area has been hampered by the lack of a suitable biological test system for investigating the action of thymus extracts.

The weight and cellular activity of lymphoid tissues and particularly the levels of blood lymphocytes in the mouse are extremely labile, fluctuating widely in response to influences which often appear trivial. It is not widely known, for example, that a characteristic lymphopenia develops in mice within minutes following such minor procedures as earmarking, tailpricking to obtain blood, or simple puncture of the skin at sham injection. This lymphopenic response is maximal after 30—60 minutes and passes off after 3—6 hours (Fig. 26) (METCALF, unpublished data). It is not related

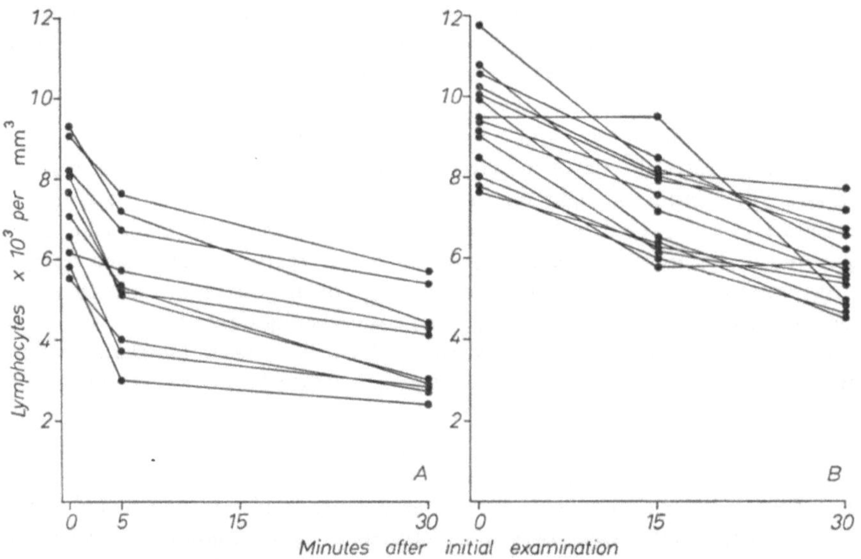

Fig. 26. Lymphopenic response in tail blood to the trauma associated with tail bleeding to perform the actual white cell counts in normal (A) and adrenalectomised (B) two months old C3H mice. Curves represent individual mice

to adrenal mediated stress responses and occurs in adrenalectomised animals. In response to more severe procedures such as sham operation or the injection of foreign material (particularly intravenously), adrenal-mediated stress reactions become superimposed on the foregoing phenomenon, producing a more lasting lymphopenia which may be followed by a lymphocytosis during wound repair. These phenomena are even more marked in neonatal animals and greatly complicate the interpretation of results following such simple procedures as the injection of thymus extract.

Absolute blood lymphocyte levels in apparently normal mice also fluctuate disturbingly from one period of the year to another. The basis for these fluctuations is very poorly understood but population density, temperature and the level of endemic infections and infestations in the mouse colony are all known to be involved. The blood lymphocyte levels of larger laboratory animals seem much less prone to fluctuation. It seems desirable that future experiments on the effects of thymus extracts be restricted to those animals in which lymphocyte levels have been standardised by procedures, such as raising the animals under germfree or pathogen free conditions or the use of small doses of whole body irradiation. Alternatively, experiments with thymus extracts may need to be restricted to large animals which have an inherently more stable lymphoid system.

Despite these depressing introductory remarks, it has been possible to demonstrate some effects of thymus extracts on the lymphoid tissues and these will now be discussed. In 1954 we made attempts to grow human leukaemic lymphocytes in a heterologous host by the injection of whole leukaemic blood into the brains of day old mice. This procedure was chosen because of the immunological tolerance of the neonatal mouse and because the brain is known to be relatively free of lymphoid cells and to support the growth of foreign tissue. It was observed that mice injected with blood from patients with chronic lymphoid leukaemia subsequently developed a lymphocytosis. It was assumed initially that the additional lymphoid cells observed in the blood might be human cells, but control experiments using sera from the same patients showed that the lymphocytosis was a response to some factor present in the chronic lymphoid leukaemic sera (METCALF, 1956).

Further experiments showed that material with a similar lymphocytosis stimulating activity was present in the sera of patients with lymphosarcoma but was not detectable in the sera of patients with acute leukaemia or acute or chronic myeloid leukaemia. Similarly, the sera from normal persons and patients with a variety of other diseases (including patients with a lymphocytosis following pertussis) also showed no lymphocytosis stimulating activity (METCALF, 1956 a).

These chance observations led to a survey being made of the lymphocytosis stimulating activity of cell free extracts of various human and mouse tissues. In the case of the mouse it was found that saline extracts of thymus tissue would produce a lymphocytosis when injected into baby mice but not extracts of lymph node, spleen, liver, kidney, lung, muscle or brain (METCALF, 1956 b). The active principle in thymus extracts was termed the lymphocytosis stimulating factor (LSF). In these experiments, organs were ground at room temperature in a pestle and mortar with silica and the organ suspension in normal (unbuffered) saline centrifuged at 3000 rpm for five minutes to remove cell debris. The mice used for injection were from a random bred colony of Hall Institute strain mice. These mice have large (8—12) litters and litter size was standardised to 6 babies of uniform size per mother, by culling out small or unhealthy babies. These baby mice were then injected intracerebrally when aged one to two days, 0.02 ml. of organ extract being injected into the left cerebral hemisphere. In most of this work the intracerebral route of injection was used, since material injected by this route in neonatal mice rapidly reaches the circulation (e.g. chicken red cells appear in the tail blood within 30 seconds). However subsequent experiments showed that thymus extracts were equally effective when injected subcutaneously or intraperitoneally. Mice tolerated intracerebrally injected material well and the mortality from the injection of a wide range of tissue extracts in these experiments averaged less than 5%.

Following the injection of thymus extracts, the baby mice slowly developed a lymphocytosis which showed its greatest height six days after injection. This lymphocytosis was superimposed on the normal increase in blood lymphocytes occurring in the first week of life (Fig. 27). Polymorph levels usually remained within control levels. By day 10 after injection, lymphocyte levels in thymus extract-injected mice were no longer higher than in control mice. The performance of absolute white cell counts required so much blood that individual mice had to be used for each time point. To circumvent this difficulty, since it had been established in the colony of mice being used that thymus extracts did not affect polymorph levels, the assay for

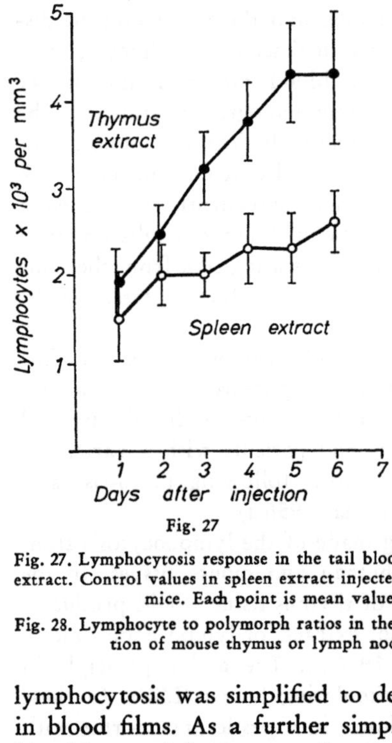

Fig. 27

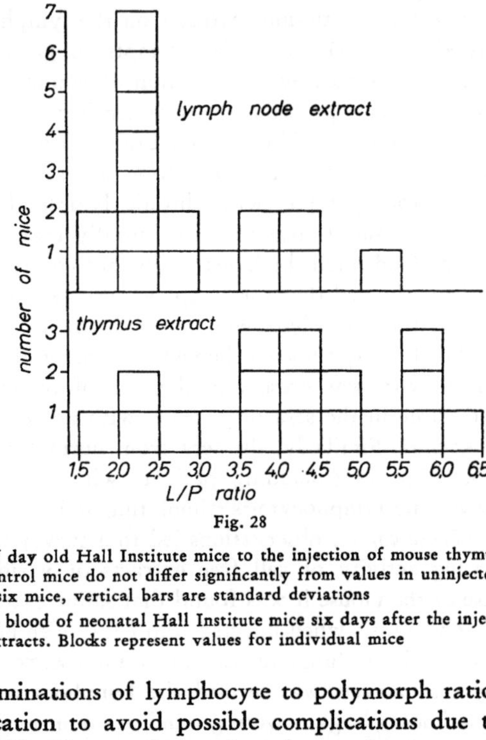

Fig. 28

Fig. 27. Lymphocytosis response in the tail blood of day old Hall Institute mice to the injection of mouse thymus extract. Control values in spleen extract injected control mice do not differ significantly from values in uninjected mice. Each point is mean value of six mice, vertical bars are standard deviations

Fig. 28. Lymphocyte to polymorph ratios in the tail blood of neonatal Hall Institute mice six days after the injection of mouse thymus or lymph node extracts. Blocks represent values for individual mice

lymphocytosis was simplified to determinations of lymphocyte to polymorph ratios in blood films. As a further simplification to avoid possible complications due to blood loss and the trauma of repeated bleedings, and since lymphocytosis was maximal at day 6, the assay procedure was limited to the determination of lymphocyte to polymorph ratios on the mice six days after the injection of test material. A typical pattern of lymphocyte to polymorph ratios in thymus extract injected and control mice at day 6 after injection is shown in Fig. 28. It will be seen that the magnitude of the lymphocytosis was not large and there was normally some overlap between the lymphocyte to polymorph ratios in thymus extract-injected and control mice. Increasing the concentration of thymus extract did not increase the level of lymphocytosis induced. However it was possible by serial dilution of thymus extracts to perform crude titrations for thymus LSF concentration in mouse thymus tissue of various ages. These titrations suggested that thymus LSF content was very low in newborn mice, high in the young adult thymus and that thymic LSF activity was low in old age.

When inbred mice were used for the assay system it was possible to show that isologous thymus extracts were capable of stimulating a similar lymphocytosis. In general however, the small litter size of the inbred mice available and the variability in size of the injected babies (with accompanying variability in lymphocyte to polymorph ratios) made inbred mice much less satisfactory than random bred mice for the assay system. When baby mice were ill, under-fed (as demonstrated by foster nursing newborn babies on nursing mothers in the second and third weeks of lactation) or given simultaneous injections of cortisone acetate, thymus extracts were unable to induce a satisfactory lymphocytosis.

The mechanisms underlying the lymphocytosis induced by thymus extracts in baby mice are unknown. Histological examination of the lymphoid tissues six days after injection gave little evidence of any change in the morphology of these tissues. The timing of the response—a slow development to maximum levels at day 6 and a fall by day 10—is compatible with a mild stimulation of lymphopoiesis but a slowly developing redistribution of preformed lymphoid cells between tissues and blood could equally well explain the observed changes.

Thymus fragments in tissue culture appeared to produce additional amounts of LSF over pre-culture content, suggesting that thymus tissue actually secretes this factor not merely serves as a repository for such material (METCALF, 1956 b). Separate assays of LSF content in thymus cortex fragments and thymus medulla tissue (with considerable contamination of cortical tissue) showed that LSF activity was associated with the medullary tissue and could not be detected in cortex extracts.

When thymus tissue, from baby mice injected with active thymus extracts, was itself tested for LSF activity 6 days later, no detectable activity could be demonstrated, suggesting some type of negative feedback control of injected LSF over the normal development of LSF in the thymus with increasing age. Thymus fragments from LSF-injected mice regained demonstrable LSF activity when maintained in tissue culture for 24 hours.

Little biochemical investigation has been carried out on the nature of thymic LSF. These studies were rendered very difficult because of the toxic properties introduced into the extracts by various biochemical treatments e.g. fat extraction or heating, for such extracts frequently produced on injection either an intense polymorph leucocytosis or death. It was established however that thymic LSF was heat labile, activity being destroyed by heating to 60° C for 15 minutes.

It was later shown that certain mice, e.g. preleukaemic AKR and C58 mice, contain what appears to be detectable levels of LSF in their sera. Assays for thymic LSF in these mice suggested that levels in the thymus in these strains may be higher than in other inbred mice (METCALF, 1959 a). When adult AKR and C58 mice were thymectomised and their sera tested for LSF activity three months later, no detectable activity was found (METCALF, 1959 a).

Subsequent to 350 r whole body irradiation, C57Bl and RF strain mice were found to have detectable lymphocytosis stimulating activity in their plasma, whereas the sera from control unirradiated mice had no similar activity (METCALF, 1959).

These experiments with thymus extracts in the baby mouse suggest that the medullary tissue of the thymus may secrete a lymphocytosis stimulating factor and that under some circumstances similar activity may be demonstrable in the serum.

A number of investigators have attempted to repeat these observations with varying success. DUPLAN, FOSCHI and MANSON (1962) reported initial success in inducing a similar type of lymphocytosis in baby mice with thymus extracts but, following some change in the baby mice being used, were unable to elicit the response. A rather similar experience was encountered by DE SOMER, DENYS and LEYTEN (1963) who initially reported the production of a lymphocytosis in normal or thymectomised mice by the injection of calf thymus but not spleen extracts. After several months' work on this phenomenon, the mice being used developed refractoriness to stimulation (DE SOMER, personal communication).

More recently CAMBLIN and BRIDGES (1964) have reported the production of a lymphocytosis in baby rats (subjected first to thymic irradiation with additional small doses of whole body irradiation, to induce a uniformly lymphopenic base line for control and injected animals) when injected with rat or rabbit thymus extracts but not when injected with heated rat thymus extract or rat spleen or brain extracts.

GREGOIRE and DUCHATEAU (1956) also reported that the injection of thymus extracts but not lymph node extracts from pigs into rats increased the weights of the lymph nodes of injected animals.

Recently KLEIN, GOLDSTEIN and WHITE (1965) have made the interesting observation that thymus extracts from either calf, rat or isologous mice increased lymph node weight and the incorporation of tritiated thymidine into lymph node DNA and of C14 glycine into lymph node protein. Increased tritiated thymidine incorporation into DNA was observed 24 hours after a single intraperitoneal injection of thymus extract containing only 7 mg. of protein but lymph node weight increase and increased glycine incorporation were not observed until after three daily injections of thymus extract. These workers reported that thymus extracts made using buffer at pH5.7 were active but those made at pH7.4 were inactive.

NAKAMOTO (1957 a) had previously reported that acid and lipide containing extracts of calf thymus produced a lymphocytosis in young rabbits. He noted that only thymus extracts from young animals were effective in producing a lymphocytosis.

As stated initially it seems possible to demonstrate the activity of thymus extracts on blood lymphocyte levels and perhaps other aspects of lymphoid organ function but the experiments have been plagued by uncontrollable variability in the test animals being used and there is an obvious need for some more reliable assay system before work along the lines of biochemical fractionation of thymus extracts can be undertaken.

That thymus tissue produces a humoral factor with activity on lymphoid organs has been successfully demonstrated indirectly by the use of thymus graft tissue in millipore diffusion chambers.

As stated earlier, neonatally thymectomised mice become severely lymphopenic. Injections of thymus extract have been reported to be ineffective in correcting this lymphopenic state (DALMASSO et al., 1963; MILLER, 1964 a). However the lymphopenia and lymphoid organ atrophy can be prevented by grafting isologous or homologous thymus tissue subcutaneously or under the kidney capsule, provided such grafts are carried out before the general health of the thymectomised mice begins to deteriorate. In such animals it is possible to demonstrate that lymphoid cells of graft origin are present and proliferating in the host lymph nodes and spleen—at least in the antigenically stimulated animal (LEUCHARS, CROSS and DAVIES, 1964; MILLER, 1965). However in the unstimulated thymectomised and thymus-grafted animals it is rather surprising that not only are most dividing cells in the host organs of host origin (MILLER, 1962 b) but all mitotic cells in the curative grafts themselves are similarly derived from the host. Similarly DALMASSO, MARTINEZ and GOOD (1964) found that when thymus grafts from C3H mice were placed in neonatally thymectomised A strain mice, the spleen recovered its normal complement of cells capable of inducing runt disease in foreign strains. However the reactivity pattern of these cells indicated that they were primarily of host not donor thymus graft origin.

This suggested that thymus grafts may correct the lymphopenic state of neonatally thymectomised animals not so much by providing cells to repopulate the host as by providing some humoral factor or a suitable environment within the graft itself enabling host lymphocyte proliferation.

Millipore diffusion chambers are plastic rings sealed by two millipore membranes to form a capsule. The millipore membranes have holes in them of varying mean diameters e.g. 0.45 μ to 0.1 μ. The smallest pore size (0.1 μ) certainly prevents the passage of cells into or out of such chambers. OSOBA and MILLER (1963; 1964), LEVEY, TRAININ and LAW (1963) and BARCLAY, WEISMAN and KAPLAN (1964) have shown that thymus tissue (either embryonic or neonatal) in millipore diffusion chambers with pore sizes varying from 0.45 μ to 0.1 μ prevents the development of a severe lymphopenic state in neonatally thymectomised animals. Blood lymphocyte levels and lymphoid organ cellularity are not completely normal, but are significantly higher than in untreated neonatally thymectomised mice of the same age. This is indisputable evidence for the existence of a humoral factor secreted by, or released from, thymus tissue which is essential in some way for the normal proliferation of lymphoid cells in the young animal.

The diffusion chamber experiments have not provided definite evidence on the thymic cell type producing this humoral factor. However it was found that thymic lymphoid cells survived very poorly in such chambers and that after a few weeks only epithelial and reticulum cell elements survived (OSOBA and MILLER, 1964). This suggests that thymic epithelial and/or reticulum cells may be responsible for humoral factor production.

The diffusion chamber experiments eliminate the possibility that host lymphoid cells actually need to enter the framework of the thymus before being able to exhibit proliferative activity, although if such cells were able to enter the thymic parenchyma they might be able to proliferate even more freely.

The consistent deficit of small lymphocytes in the lymphoid follicles of thymectomised mice has raised the suggestion that thymic humoral factor, in addition to stimulating primitive lymphocyte proliferation may also encourage or be necessary for the *maturation* of these cells to small lymphocytes. This is supported by the finding that despite general lymphoid organ atrophy, the number of primitive lymphoid cells appears to be near normal in the lymphoid tissues of thymectomised animals, suggesting the existence of some sort of maturation arrest. This suggestion that thymic humoral factor may have a maturation effect on lymphoid cells was raised earlier in the discussion of the regulation of lymphopoiesis in the thymus itself, but until experimental systems can be devised for observing and measuring the rates of maturation in lymphoid cells, this action of thymic humoral factor must remain speculative.

Most of the studies described so far on the effects of thymus extracts or thymus tissue in diffusion chambers have been made in very young animals. In another series of experiments, MILLER (1962 b) and MILLER, DOAK and CROSS (1963) have demonstrated that similar processes can occur in the adult animal. If adult thymectomy is combined with whole body irradiation a lymphopenic state can be induced which is more severe and develops more rapidly than that following thymectomy alone. Following a dose of 350 r irradiation (or 850 r combined with a resuscitating intravenous injection of isologous bone marrow) thymectomised animals have been shown to be very slow to recover actively lymphopoietic tissues and again there is a characteristic lymphopenia and a deficit of small lymphocytes in the spleen lymphoid follicles and lymph nodes in such animals. Thymus grafting of irradiated thymectomised mice is followed by regeneration of the host lymphoid organs. These "curative" thymus grafts may be from either isologous or homologous donors but, unlike the situation in the neonatal animal where the homologous thymus graft is permanently accepted by the animal, the curative homologous thymus graft in the adult recipient is rapidly broken down and destroyed within 10 days by the host lymphoid tissues which the homologous graft has been responsible for restoring. In a sense, this homologous thymus graft has been a "biological time bomb", being disrupted by the very tissues it has restored (MILLER, 1964). This experiment suggested that in the adult thymectomised irradiated animal, thymic humoral factor may need only to be present for a very short period to restore the proliferative activity of the host lymphoid tissues. This question has recently been explored directly by MILLER (1965) who resected thymus grafts at varying intervals after implantation. The results indicated that thymus grafts need only to be present for a few days in order to restore some degree of host lymphoid tissue activity.

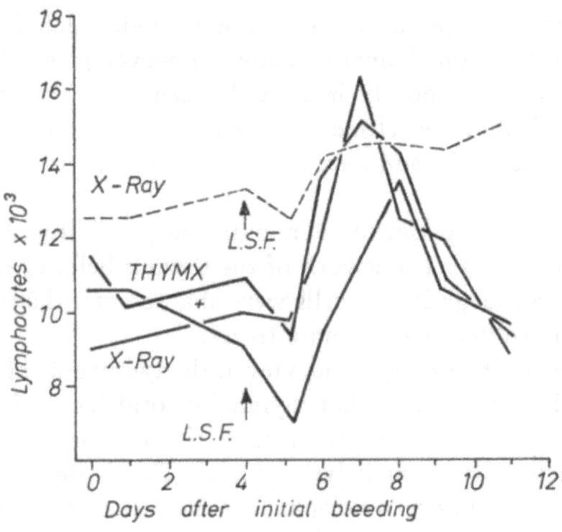

Fig. 29. Lymphocytosis response in adult thymectomised and irradiated (450 r) C57Bl mice to the injection of C57Bl thymus extract. Each line represents mean values for four mice

Previous to this work it was shown (METCALF, 1959) that thymus extracts when injected into adult thymectomised and irradiated mice produce a temporary lymphocytosis (Fig. 29) and this phenomenon in adult thymectomised and irradiated animals has recently been confirmed by CAMBLIN and BRIDGES (1964, personal communication).

As distinct from this work on the effects of thymus extracts in neonatal animals and adult thymectomised animals, many experiments in our laboratory have failed to demonstrate any effect of thymus extracts in normal adult mice. There have been isolated reports from time to time (COMSA, 1956; NAKAMOTO, 1957 a) that thymus extracts produced a lymphocytosis in adult animals and that thymus extracts induced a rise in thymic lymphoid mitotic activity (TELKKA and TIER, 1955). However we have been unable to observe any effect of isologous or homologous thymus extracts in adult C3H, C57Bl or AKR mice, given by various routes and with various injection schedules, on blood lymphocyte levels or on lymphoid organ weights, histological appearances or mitotic indices. These negative results are confirmed by a failure to observe any significant changes in the lymphoid organs of adult mice bearing massive amounts of thymus graft tissue.

Our conclusions to date from this work are that it may only be possible to demonstrate thymic humoral factor stimulation of lymphoid tissues in stituations where the cellularity of these tissues is sub-normal, for example in the neonatal animal or in the adult thymectomised or thymectomised, irradiated animal. It may be that the lymphoid tissues of the normal adult animal are proliferating at a maximum (or optimal) rate determined by other control mechanisms in the body (e.g. the level of adrenal corticosteroids, and the level of antigenic stimulation) and cannot readily be further stimulated by additional amounts of thymic humoral factor. However the recent positive results of KLEIN, GOLDSTEIN and WHITE (1965) in adult animals using thymus extracts made at pH 5.7 and the negative results obtained with extracts made at pH 7.4 suggest that inhibitors may be present in simple thymus extracts prepared by most workers and a final decision on whether or not normal adult animals can be shown to be responsive to stimulation by thymus extracts may need to await further biochemical purification and concentration of the active principle in thymus extracts.

Summary

Thymectomy, particularly in the young animal or combined with whole body irradiation in adult animals, leads to the development of severe lymphopenia and lymphoid organ atrophy in which the cell type affected most severely is the small lymphocyte. Thymus grafts correct this lymphopenic state as do thymus grafts in cell tight millipore diffusion chambers. Thymus extracts have been shown to induce a lymphocytosis in neonatal animals and in adult thymectomised and thymectomised irradiated animals. The thymic humoral factor may be secreted by the epithelial and reticulum cell elements of the thymus, primarily by those located in the medulla.

Chapter 6

The Thymus and Immune Responses

1. Effect of the Thymus on Immune Responses

As previously described, thymic lymphoid proliferative activity appears to be independent of antigenic stimulation and characteristically the thymus cortex lacks lymphoid follicles and germinal centres and contains very few plasma cells. From this it might be assumed that the thymus itself is not actively involved in local immune responses. This has been confirmed by direct studies on the production of antibodies by thymus tissue and on the immune competence of thymic lymphoid cells.

Thymus tissue does not appear to form antibodies *in vivo* (BJORNEBOE, GORMSEN and LUNDQUIST, 1947) or *in vitro* (THORBECKE and KEUNING, 1953) in response to antigen injections. THORBECKE and COHEN (1964) observed that immunisation *in vivo* failed to stimulate the *in vitro* synthesis of gammaglobulin by neonatal rabbit thymus tissue unlike with other lymphoid tissues, although some gammaglobulin synthesis was demonstrated by adult rabbit thymus tissue. VAN FURTH (cited by THORBECKE and COHEN, 1964) has also shown the acquisition by adult human thymus tissue of some capacity to form gamma and beta 2A globulins. Beta 2 macroglobulin production (the protein produced in primary immune responses) has not been observed in normal thymus tissue.

In contrast to this inability of thymus tissue to exhibit primary responses to antigenic stimulation, it has been found possible to transfer secondary responses to antigenic stimulation by the injection of thymus cells from immunised animals. Thus DIXON, WEIGLE and ROBERTS (1957) in the rabbit, and STONER and HALE (1955) in mice have transferred responses to bovine serum albumin and tetanus toxoid, and THORBECKE and COHEN (1964) demonstrated transfer of secondary responses to bovine gammaglobulin with rabbit thymus cells.

These cell transfer studies, in which antigen and antigen-carrying macrophages are also transferred, need repetition using the modern technique of allotypic identification of the antibody gammaglobulin being produced in the recipient animal before constituting proof that the injected thymic cells are actually the cells producing the antibody.

Recently MOLLER (1965) has used a modification of the Jerne plaque technique as a direct test of antibody forming capacity of various cells. Using a primary injection of a bacterial antigen in mice, he found that in most mice few or no antibody forming cells were present in the thymus. However, in occasional mice, the thymus contained large numbers of antibody forming cells. The histological structure of such thymus glands needs investigation to eliminate the possible presence of abnormal lymphoid follicles which might contain the active cells.

Cell transfer studies assessing immunological competence by the ability of injected cells to provoke graft versus host reactions (e.g. parental cells in F_1 hybrid mice or rat cells in mice) have also demonstrated the limited effectiveness of thymus cells compared with spleen or lymph node cells (THORBECKE and COHEN, 1964; BILLINGHAM and SILVERS, 1964). In general, much larger numbers of thymus cells need to be transferred than spleen or lymph node cells to demonstrate any activity. WARNER

(1964) has shown in the chicken thymus that some thymic cells will produce chorio-allantoic pox in the Simonsen-type response in chick embryos and further that the number of pock-producing cells in the thymus increases with increasing age. However, the chicken thymus may be a special case, for it seems likely that the cells provoking the membrane response are present in the medulla, and it is known that in the chicken the amount of thymic medullary tissue increases with advancing age. In mammals the possibility exists also that the limited immunological activity which is observed with thymic cell suspensions may be due to medullary lymphoid cells or to cells of the peripheral blood trapped in the organ when it is removed for testing.

If little immune reactivity appears to occur within the thymus itself, the thymus does have a profound influence on the immune reactivity of other lymphoid organs. This thymic influence was most clearly demonstrated by an analysis of the immune competence of neonatally thymectomised animals. As has been alluded to earlier, the initial studies on the fate of mice thymectomised in the first 24 hours of life indicated that after a period of apparent good health, lasting several weeks to a few months, body growth ceased in such mice. The mice became sick and developed a hunched posture with ruffled fur. They lost weight and most finally died within two to three months of operation. This "runting syndrome", as it was termed, was associated with lymphopenia and lymphoid organ atrophy. Histologically there was no obvious evidence of infection in the mice although some mice did have necrotic lesions in the liver suggesting viral infection. In neonatally thymectomised rats, a more obvious susceptibility to infections was noted for many animals developed mediastinal abscesses and bronchopneumonia (Azar, 1964). It seemed likely that the cause of death in many neonatally thymectomised mice and rats was overwhelming infection but direct attempts to isolate pathogenic organisms met with little success. East et al. (1963) reported the isolation of MHV-1 hepatitis virus from neonatally thymectomised mice showing wasting and we have observed in occasional neonatally thymectomised mice an activation of latent infection with Eperythrozoon coccoides, resulting in haemolytic anaemia. However these two isolations are exceptional and most animals as yet have not been found to contain any obvious pathogenic organisms. Azar (1964) reported that neonatally thymectomised rats maintained on antibiotics exhibited a reduced incidence of sepsis and wasting.

The real proof of the infectious aetiology of runting and death in neonatally thymectomised animals came from a study of the fate of neonatally thymectomised mice reared in germfree conditions by McIntire, Sell and Miller (1964) and Wilson, Sjodin and Bealmar (1964). Both groups reported that when mice were raised under germfree conditions, neonatal thymectomy did not cause wasting or premature death although such mice were still unable to reject foreign skin grafts. Germfree mice transferred to conventional animal rooms at intervals after neonatal thymectomy had an incidence of post-thymectomy runting and death intermediate between germfree and conventional neonatally thymectomised animals. The conclusion seems firmly established that neonatal thymectomy causes death in animals because it renders them more susceptible to endogenous infectious agents in their normal environment.

The subnormal resistance to infectious agents of neonatally thymectomised mice and rats suggested that it should be possible in such animals to demonstrate other immunological deficiencies. Miller (1961; 1962) demonstrated that neonatally thymectomised mice would tolerate skin grafts from mice of other strains and even from rats. In addition these mice showed diminished agglutinin responses to Salmonella typhi H antigen.

Similarly JANKOVIC, WAKSMAN and ARNASON (1962) found that neonatal thymectomy in rats markedly impaired delayed hypersensitivity and Arthus reactivity following the injection of bovine serum albumin with adjuvant. Such neonatally thymectomised rats also failed to develop significant titres of precipitin or haemagglutinating antibody. ARNASON et al. (1962) demonstrated that neonatal thymectomy in rats reduced the degree of tuberculin sensitivity following a single injection of tubercle bacilli in oil and rejection of skin homografts was delayed. The susceptibility to development of adjuvant arthritis following neonatal thymectomy was not affected, but blood lymphocyte levels following adjuvant administration were strikingly lower in thymectomised rats than in control rats.

GOOD et al. (1962) reported that neonatal thymectomy in mice decreased immune responses to T2 phage and allowed acceptance of skin and tumour grafts across minor histocompatibility barriers between different mouse strains. Neonatal thymectomy was also found to allow skin graft survival across the major H2 histocompatibility barrier in mice and survival of male skin grafts in female C57Bl mice. Lymphoid and spleen cells from neonatally thymectomised mice of parental strain were unable to produce splenomegaly in young F_1 hybrid recipients. GOOD et al. (1962) also found that neonatal thymectomy rendered F_1 hybrid mice more susceptible to induction of runting and death following the injection of parental spleen cells.

The decreased immunological responsiveness of the neonatally thymectomised animal does not apply to all antigens and it has been reported that the responses of such mice to ferritin, haemocyanin, T4 phage and Pneumococcus Type III polysaccharide are normal (LAW et al., 1964; HUMPHREY, PARROTT and EAST, 1964). Similarly DEFENDI, ROOSA and KOPROWSKI (1964) and TING and LAW (1965) have shown that neonatally thymectomised hamsters and mice infected with polyoma virus develop significant levels of anti-viral antibody but are unable to produce the cellular type response against the polyoma-induced host cell antigen.

In parallel with this patchy and variable loss of immunological competence, the sera of neonatally thymectomised animals have been found to have reduced, normal or even raised gammaglobulin levels [the latter, particularly in the presence of pyogenic infections (AZAR, 1964)]. AZAR (1964) also reported that beta 2A globulin levels were elevated in neonatally thymectomised rats, although ARNASON, DE VAUX ST. CYR and GRABAR (1963) reported in neonatally thymectomised rats an absence or deficiency of an immunoglobulin designated B 2A globulin.

HUMPHREY, PARROT and EAST (1964) made a detailed study of gammaglobulin levels and immune responses in neonatally thymectomised C3H/Bi and (C57Bl × C3H/Bi)F_1 mice. Thymectomised mice were found to recover from the physiological hypogammaglobulinaemia of early life more slowly than intact mice, but ultimately developed near-normal gammaglobulin levels. Increased gamma 1A globulin levels were observed in some thymectomised mice surviving longer than 7 weeks. Macroglobulin (gamma 1M) was detected in some of the mice exhibiting normal amounts of gammaglobulin. Plasma albumin turnover was normal in thymectomised mice but plasma gammaglobulin turnover was accelerated in most of the thymectomised mice examined (half life 76 hours in thymectomised mice, versus 128 hours in control mice). No evidence was obtained in neonatally thymectomised mice for the presence of autoantibodies against red cells (direct Coombs test) or for antinuclear or anticytoplasmic antibodies (guinea pig liver sections were treated with sera from thymectomised mice and later treated with fluorescein congugated rabbit anti-mouse gammaglobulin).

The influence of the thymus in early life on immune responses has also been demonstrated in neonatal rabbits. ARCHER and PIERCE (1961) and ARCHER et al. (1962) demonstrated that thymectomy at 0—5 days of age in New Zealand albino rabbits reduced precipitin production to BSA when the animals were tested at 7—8 weeks of age. When thymectomy was delayed until 5—7 days of age, no depression of the subsequent response to BSA was observed. Neonatally thymectomised rabbits were also found to produce less neutralising antibody to T2 phage (GOOD et al., 1962). However neonatal thymectomy did not affect the speed of rejection of skin grafts from Dutch rabbits.

As described previously, subcutaneous or kidney subcapsular isologous thymus grafts, if placed in neonatally thymectomised mice before serious clinical illness has become apparent, will prevent lymphocyte depletion in the lymphoid tissues and prevent body weight loss and death. Tests for immunological competence in such grafted mice have revealed a near-normal capacity to synthethise antibodies to all antigens tested and these grafted mice reject foreign skin grafts within normal rejection times (MILLER, 1962). In neonatally thymectomised animals it is also possible to restore immunological competence and prevent death by grafting thymus tissue from homologous donors (e.g. C3H thymus grafts in strain C57Bl mice). Being neonatal animals these mice permanently accept the foreign thymus graft and thereafter also will tolerate other tissue grafts (e.g. skin grafts) from the same donor strain (MILLER, 1962 b; DALMASSO et al., 1963).

However with this exception it has been a universal finding that when thymus grafts restore the immunological competence of neonatally thymectomised mice, the mice retain their own pattern of immunological responsiveness. Specifically they do *not* acquire the immunological responsiveness of the thymus donor strain. It seems therefore that the thymus does not *instruct* lymphoid cells in the sense of determining to which antigenic patterns they will develop an immunological response, instead the thymus graft in a neonatally thymectomised animal merely makes it possible for host lymphoid cells to *initiate* those immune responses which they should normally have been capable of exhibiting.

The initial analysis of neonatally thymectomised mice protected by thymus grafts indicated that most of the lymphoid cells in these "cured" animals were actually of host origin. This raised the likelihood that in this situation the thymus may merely have been producing a humoral factor which was necessary to allow the non-thymic lymphoid cells to respond to antigenic stimulation.

However DALMASSO et al. (1963) and MILLER (1964 a) reported that the injection of saline extracts of thymus into neonatally thymectomised mice did not prevent wasting and did not restore immune competence. JANKOVIC, WAKSMAN and ARNASON (1962) also reported that the injection of thymus or spleen cell homogenates did not improve the immune reactivity of neonatally thymectomised rats.

Proof that the thymus influences immune responses by means of a humoral factor was obtained by OSOBA and MILLER (1963, 1964) and independently by LEVEY,

Trainin and Law (1963) and Law et al. (1964). Osoba and Miller implanted intraperitoneally millipore diffusion chambers containing embryonic thymus tissue in (CBA × T6)F_1 mice, 7 days after neonatal thymectomy. The subsequent growth of these mice was normal and when they were challenged later with foreign skin grafts, most mice rejected the foreign grafts within the normal rejection period. The production of normal titres of haemagglutinin to sheep red cells was also demonstrable in neonatally thymectomised mice bearing millipore diffusion chambers with thymus tissue but not in mice grafted with empty diffusion chambers. Similarly, Law et al. (1964) reported that thymus graft tissue in millipore diffusion chambers in neonatally thymectomised C3H and DBA strain mice restored the haemolysin response to the primary injection of sheep red cells as effectively as did subcutaneous thymus grafts.

Law et al. (1964 a) have demonstrated an interesting alternative source of thymic humoral factor for restoring immune competence in thymectomised animals. One strain (SV10) of polyoma virus has been demonstrated to induce a high incidence of epithelial cell thymic tumours in mice. Pieces of these neoplasms were injected into (C57Bl × C3Hf/Lw)F_1 mice 3 days after neonatal thymectomy. The tumour tissue grew to palpable size but then regressed. When these recipient mice were examined subsequently, 71% were found to have grown normally although they were still slightly lymphopenic. These mice were found capable of developing a normal antibody response to injected sheep red cells. It seems possible that the neoplastic thymic epithelial cells remained functional and were able to secrete sufficient humoral factor to restore immunological reactivity in the thymectomised host lymphoid tissues.

These findings on the existence and effectiveness of a thymic humoral factor in restoring the cellularity and immune reactivity of lymphoid tissues clearly prove that the thymus does not function simply as a factory producing competent lymphoid cells for use by other lymphoid organs in immune responses. It remains possible however that cell production and seeding by the thymus might occur and if so, this would represent an accessory thymic function to humoral regulation of the lymphoid organs by the thymus. In the data so far reported on thymectomised animals treated with thymus grafts in diffusion chambers, there are suggestions that such treatment may greatly improve the animals but may not restore them to full normality. Such studies need to be carried out for longer time intervals than have been done so far to determine whether or not lymphocyte numbers ever achieve normal levels, and particularly whether in later life a lymphoid deficient state may not subsequently recur in the continued absence of any cell delivery from the thymus tissue. Until such long term studies are made it cannot be claimed that lymphocyte delivery from the thymus is of no significance for the full functional efficiency of the non thymic lymphoid tissues.

Jerne, Nordin and Henry (1963) introduced a plaque technique which makes possible the demonstration of 19S antibody production by single cells in response to the injection of sheep red cells. Following the injection of sheep red cells in normal animals, there is a rapid proliferation of cells in the spleen which are capable of forming haemolytic plaques with sheep red cells and complement. This proliferative response reaches its peak at 4—5 days and coincides with the peak of 19S antibody production in such animals. It has been shown by Moller (personal communication) that during the immune response to sheep red cells, the number of plaque forming cells in normal mouse spleen doubles every 5—7 hours—the rate of increase of these cells depending in part on the dose of antigen used.

Recently FRIEDMAN (1965) has obtained data which indicate more precisely the exact influence of the thymus on antibody formation. Using the JERNE plaque technique he studied the behaviour of haemolytic plaque-forming cells in the spleen following primary immunisation with sheep red blood cells. Neonatal NIH albino white mice were subjected to thymectomy or sham operation and at 6 weeks of age the mice were injected intraperitoneally with sheep red cells. Haemolysin titres at 4 days were only 1 : 31 in the thymectomised mice compared with titres of 1 : 428 in control mice. At day 0, thymectomised spleens were only 100 mg. compared with sham operated spleen weights of approximately 200 mg. After immunisation, sham operated spleen weights doubled by day 4 but in thymectomised mice little weight change was observed. At day 0, 0.08 plaque forming cells per 10^6 spleen cells were present in thymectomised mice versus 0.42 per 10^6 in sham operated mice. In both types of mice the number of plaque forming cells rose following immunisation, but the rise was more rapid and reached a far higher peak number in control mice (1500 per 10^6 spleen cells by day 2) than in thymectomised mice (2.1 per 10^6 spleen cells by day 2). As judged by the diameter of the plaques, those plaque forming cells which were present in thymectomised spleens were producing as much antibody as individual cells in control spleens. Data obtained by MILLER (1965) confirm these observations of FRIEDMAN on the effect of thymectomy on the plaque-forming cell response to sheep red cells and also indicate that thymus grafts restore to normal the rate of plaque-forming cell increase following the injection of sheep red cells. The longer the thymus grafts were left in the recipient thymectomised mice, the greater the number of plaque-forming cells present a peak response to the antigen. Three to four weeks after thymus grafting, the neonatally thymectomised animals gave normal plaque-forming responses with sheep red cells.

It is quite apparent that, following neonatal thymectomy, not only is the size of the starting population (day 0) of plaque-forming cells reduced but the rate of replication of these cells is greatly diminished following stimulation by sheep red cells. On the other hand the amount of antibody produced by individual cells does not appear to be depressed by thymectomy.

The morphology of plaque-forming cells is still a little uncertain but these cells are probably members of the plasma cell series, ranging from primitive plasma cells to relatively mature plasma cells.

It should be emphasised that the accumulation of plaque-forming cells in the spleen during an immune response is an exponential one. This indicates that the total number of these cells is increased by cellular *proliferation* rather than by the simple importation of cells from some other site. The data of FRIEDMAN and MILLER clearly indicate that one of the influences of the thymus on immune responses must be to accelerate the rate at which plasma cell precursors proliferate following antigenic stimulation.

In the immune response to the injection of an antigen such as sheep red cells, a *dual* response occurs in the lymphoid tissues. Not only is there a wave of proliferation in cells of the plasma cell series, but there is also increased lymphopoiesis leading to enlargement of lymphoid follicles and a lymphocytosis in the blood. So far as is known, true lymphoid cells—particularly small lymphocytes—are not capable of forming haemolytic plaques. This would suggest that the increased lymphopoiesis and accumulation of small lymphocytes which follow antigenic stimulation are a separate facet of the immune response. The fact that germinal centre mitotic activity and the number of small lymphocytes in lymphoid tissues is severely reduced by thymectomy would then suggest that the thymus affects both facets of the immune response—the rate of plasma cell proliferation and also the rate of antigen-stimulated primitive lymphocyte proliferation and maturation to small lymphocytes.

Since thymus grafts in diffusion chambers restore to normal the antibody forming capacity of thymectomised animals and to some extent at least, the morphology of the lymphoid germinal centres and follicles, it seems reasonable to conclude that thymic humoral factor mediates both effects of the thymus. In more precise terms thymic humoral factor appears to accelerate the *rate of proliferation* of those particular primitive plasma cells and lymphoid cells which are stimulated to proliferate following exposure to the antigen to which they are competent to respond (Fig. 30).

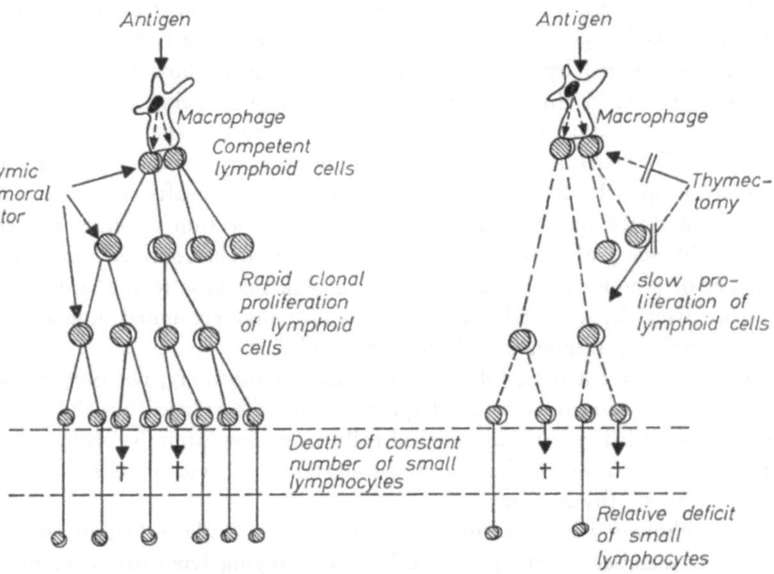

Fig. 30. Schematic representation of the action of thymic humoral factor in accelerating the proliferative response of competent lymphoid cells to macrophage processed antigen. Following thymectomy, the proliferative response is reduced leading, in the face of the death or loss of a constant number of small lymphocytes, to a relative deficit of small lymphocytes

It is not known whether thymic humoral factor stimulates the proliferation of these types of cell in the *absence* of specific antigen. It is true that unimmunised (day 0) thymectomised mice have fewer plaque-forming cells capable of haemolysing sheep red cells than do sham operated mice but it is believed that, in this system, low level antigenic stimulation of these clones of cells is occurring continuously in normal life, possibly due to stimulation by cross reacting bacterial antigens.

Dalmasso, Martinez and Good (1964) demonstrated that neonatal thymectomy reduced the spleen content of cells (presumably lymphoid) capable of initiating graft-versus-host runt disease in foreign neonatal recipients. This again could be interpreted as indicating that prior to cell transfer, the competent cells concerned had been unable to proliferate normally in the donor thymectomised animal in the absence of thymic humoral factor.

An interesting example of the *beneficial* effects of neonatal thymectomy in reducing immune responses was provided by ROWE, BLACK and LEVEY (1963), and EAST, PARROTT and SEAMER (1964). Lymphocytic choriomeningitis (LCM) virus infection of adult mice produces a fatal disease but neonatally-infected mice survive with a persistent viraemia because they are immunologically immature and develop tolerance to the virus. Death after LCM virus infection of adult mice is believed by HOTCHIN (1962) to result from an immune reaction of the host to the virus rather than from direct cytopathic effects of the virus on the host cell. In the experiments of EAST, PARROTT and SEAMER, Swiss albino TO mice were thymectomised at less than 24 hours of age and injected intracerebrally with LCM virus at 2 weeks of age. Only 20% of such mice died, which was little more than the 12% of control neonatally thymectomised mice dying in the same period. By contrast, 75% of intact 2 weeks old mice injected with LCM virus died within 12 days of infection. The thymectomised mice were shown to have supported LCM virus proliferation and to have been viraemic when tested subsequently.

Before leaving the subject of the effect of neonatal thymectomy on immune responses, reference should be made to two rare conditions in man which may be the equivalent of neonatal thymectomy in animals.

In 1950, GLANZMANN and RINIKER described a type of agammaglobulinaemia in infants in which there was an associated lymphopenia and extreme atrophy of the peripheral lymphoid tissues, and other examples of this desease have now been reported (GOOD, MARTINEZ and GABRIELSEN, 1964). These patients are extremely susceptible to infections and die in the first two years of life. The thymus is extremely atrophic in such cases and little more than a few epithelial and stromal elements of abnormal morphology may be found. The condition may well represent a situation in which the thymus fails to develop, leading in effect to a neonatally thymectomised state, with resulting lymphoid atrophy and depressed immune responses.

GOOD (1954) and MACLEAN et al. (1956) reported the association of acquired agammaglobulinaemia with benign epithelial thymic tumours and a number of similar cases have been reported subsequently. Possibly these also represent states equivalent to functional thymectomy for these patients exhibited hypersusceptibility to infections.

As has been seen from the preceding discussion, there is strong evidence that in neonatal life, the thymus plays an essential role in the development by the animal of full immunological competence. This raises the obvious question of whether this thymic function persits throughout adult life.

Neonatally thymectomised mice may be saved from sickness and early death not only by thymus grafting, but also by the injection of isologous *adult* spleen or lymph node cells. Thymus cell suspensions can be used to save such mice (LAW et al., 1964 a; MILLER, 1964) but appear (particularly neonatal thymic cells) to be much less efficient than spleen cells and massive numbers of thymic cells must be injected to save the animals. Further, although thymus cells may save the thymectomised recipients from death, the restoration of immune competence by thymic cells is very incomplete (DALMASSO et al., 1963). However neonatally thymectomised mice injected with adult spleen cells give normal antibody responses and reject foreign grafts within normal time intervals (MILLER, 1964 a).

In similar studies EAST and PARROTT (1964) found that AKR thymus grafts either subcutaneously or under the kidney capsule prevented wasting and lymphocyte depletion in neonatally thymectomised C3H/Bi mice. Multiple subcutaneous doses of 30×10^6 syngeneic (C3H) thymus cells also allowed normal growth and development but a single intravenous injection of $5-50 \times 10^6$ thymus cells was ineffective. Syngeneic adult spleen cells were more effective than thymus cells in protecting neonatally thymectomised animals and a single intravenous dose of 30×10^6 cells saved mice from wasting. However spleen cells from neonatally thymectomised donors did not prevent wasting. Pooled serum from adult C3H mice given in doses of 0.5 ml. intraperitoneally twice weekly for up to 7 weeks did not prevent wasting and death in neonatally thymectomised mice.

Similarly AISENBERG, WILKES and WAKSMAN (1962) found that adult homologous spleen cells were able to produce severe runt disease in rats thymectomised at 3 days of age as rapidly as in normal animals, suggesting that immune reactivity of *adult* cells was not dependent on a thymic humoral influence.

These findings suggested to some that whilst the lymphoid tissue of neonatal animals may need a thymic influence to exhibit normal immune responses, adult lymphoid tissues no longer need such an influence and thus it seemed to these workers that the thymus might not exert any immunological function in adult life. Actually the experimental observations on which this reasoning was based may not be quite correct for although neonatally thymectomised animals injected with adult cells do well initially, if such animals are kept for long enough their condition ultimately deteriorates and after six months they begin to die prematurely (LAW, personal communication). This latter observation would suggest that adult lymphoid cells may function well in the absence of the thymus, but only for a limited period, after which unless thymus tissue is present the functional activity of these cells (or their number) declines.

Suggestions that the thymus might continue to affect immune responses in adult life were obtained by GOOD et al. (1962) and MARTINEZ et al. (1962 a) whose results indicated that if foreign antigens were weak, adult thymectomy might exert a sufficiently depressing influence on host immune responses to allow observable differences between thymectomised and sham operated control mice. Thymectomy in C3H mice at 30 days of age allowed permanent acceptance of Ce strain skin homografts in 63% of mice. Both C3H and Ce strain mice belong to the same $H\text{-}2^k$ histocompatibility subgroup so that the antigen differences between these strains are minor. However control C3H mice regularly rejected skin homografts from Ce strain mice.

Where strong H-2 histocompatibility differences existed e.g. between $(A \times C3H)F_1$ and C3H mice, even adult splenectomy combined with thymectomy did not result in any survival of skin homografts. Similarly in C57Bl mice, adult thymectomy did not prevent rejection of male skin grafts by female mice responding to the Y chromosome-dependent antigens.

Similar results were obtained when tumour homografts were employed as the challenge system. Adult thymectomy of DBA/2 mice allowed these mice to accept homografts of Balb/C multiple myeloma tissue (both H-2d) but adult thymectomy of C3H mice did not allow acceptance of mammary tumour transplants from strain A mice (C3H mice are H-2[k] whereas A strain mice are H-2[a]).

Martinez et al. (1962) also demonstrated that adult thymectomy of F_1 mice increased their susceptibility to, and accelerated the course of, graft-versus-host reactions produced by the injection of spleen cells from parental strain donors, and Dalmasso, et al. (1963) demonstrated that thymectomy as late as 35 days of age reduced the spleen content of cells capable of eliciting a graft-versus-host reaction in F_1 strain recipients. Further it was noted that the longer the adult thymectomised mice were left before testing, the greater the degree of depletion of the spleen content of immunologically active cells.

Direct evidence has now been obtained that the thymic influence on antibody production persists in adult life. It has been observed repeatedly that thymectomy in adult life has no effect, or only a minimal effect, on the immune responsiveness of such animals when tests are carried out immediately after operation (Harris, Rhoads and Stokes, 1948; Maclean et al., 1956; Fichtelius, Laurell and Philipsson, 1961). However Miller (1962 a) demonstrated that if adult thymectomy in mice was combined with 350 r whole body irradiation, such mice exhibited depressed haemagglutinin responses to sheep red cells and a delayed rejection time of homologous skin grafts. When the dose of whole body irradiation was increased to 850 r, an even greater depression of immune responses was observed (Miller, Doak and Cross, 1963; Cross, Leuchars and Miller, 1964). When high dosages of irradiation were used, the irradiated mice needed the injection of isologous bone marrow, liver or spleen cells to allow survival, but whereas the adult spleen cell injections also restored immune competence, neither the adult bone marrow cells nor the foetal liver cells restored immune competence unless the recipients were also grafted with thymus tissue. Mice given 40×10^6 bone marrow cells without thymus grafting exhibited only slight restoration of immune competence. Spleen cells from neonatally thymectomised donors were unable to restore immune competence. Where thymus grafts and bone marrow cells were used to restore immune competence in lethally irradiated thymectomised adult recipients, the cells repopulating the thymus grafts and constituting the major proliferative population in the host lymphoid organs were demonstrated to have come not from the donor thymus graft but the donor bone marrow cells.

A similar effect of whole body irradiation combined with adult thymectomy in depressing immune responses was reported by Globerson and Feldman (1964) using challenge with foreign tumour cell transplants as the index of immune competence. Normal C3H mice were able to reject transplants of a chemically induced sarcoma of C57Bl strain mice. However after 550 r whole body irradiation, approximately 40% of C3H mice permitted the progressive proliferation of these sarcoma cells. Virtually all C3H mice subjected to both thymectomy in adult life and 550 r whole body irradiation allowed progressive growth of the C57Bl tumour cells. A similar result was observed in the reciprocal combination of challenge of C57Bl thymectomised and irradiated mice with a C3H sarcoma. In thymectomised irradiated C3H mice, the grafting of neonatal C3H thymus grafts restored the ability of the animals to reject C57Bl tumour transplants. Interestingly, C57Bl thymus grafts also restored the ability of most of the C3H mice to reject C57Bl sarcoma transplants. This result indicates again that the thymic stromal elements do not dictate the pattern of immune reactivity to be expressed by the host lymphoid cells—but merely activate these cells to express their own genetically determined reactivity patterns.

In these experiments it was also observed that thymus grafts from 1 month old donors were less effective in restoring immune competence than neonatal thymus grafts—an effect probably resulting from the superior growth capacity of neonatal thymus grafts, as described earlier.

The situation with respect to bone marrow cells and immune competence is of considerable interest. As was stated earlier, bone marrow cells can repopulate the thymus of irradiated mice, (FORD and MICKLEM, 1963) and the bone marrow is the probable source of the cells repopulating the thymus throughout normal life. In the irradiated animal, injected bone marrow cells can also be observed in the repopulating tissues of the spleen and lymph nodes. However it has been shown clearly (MILLER, DOAK and CROSS, 1963; CROSS, LEUCHARS and MILLER, 1964; MILLER et al., 1964) that bone marrow cells from normal adult mice if given alone, cannot restore the cellularity or the immune reactivity of the lymphoid tissues of neonatally thymectomised mice or adult thymectomised irradiated mice. Paradoxically, bone marrow cells must be given along with thymus grafts to lethally irradiated thymectomised mice to permit survival—but here the bone marrow cells are primarily required to provide erythropoietic and myelopoietic tissue.

It seems likely that the bone marrow does not contain cells of the type present in adult lymph node and spleen which can seed in the tissues of neonatally thymectomised animals and restore immune responses without thymic intervention. Either bone marrow cells must first enter the thymus and be modified by the thymus before reseeding to the tissues, as proposed by HARRIS and FORD (1964), or the bone marrow cells may seed in the lymphoid tissues but need activation by thymic humoral factor before being capable of responding to antigenic stimulation. This latter possibility seems more likely in view of the finding of MILLER (1965) that when bone marrow cells were injected intravenously to lethally irradiated adult thymectomised mice carrying a foreign thymus graft under the kidney capsule, immune competence was restored and the animals rejected the curative foreign thymus graft, yet no mitoses of donor marrow type were observed in the thymus graft. Similarly bone marrow from thymectomised irradiated donor mice injected into irradiated recipients allowed homologous skin transplant rejection by the recipient, provided the recipient's thymus was still present (CROSS, LEUCHARS and MILLER, 1964). This concept of a pool of "unprimed" lymphoid precursor cells in the bone marrow which can be activated by thymic humoral factor will be discussed in more detail later.

The time sequence of the restoration of immune competence in adult thymectomised irradiated mice indicates that the thymic influence need only be present for a few days to restore (temporarily at least) immune competence.

It seems likely that the more marked effect of adult thymectomy on immune responses when combined with whole body irradiation results from the destruction by the irradiation of pre-existing immunologically competent lymphoid cells. In this regard it has been shown by both MILLER, and FELDMAN and GLOBERSON, that regeneration of the lymphoid tissues following irradiation is slower and less complete when the host is thymectomised.

This action of irradiation in destroying lymphoid tissues, necessitating subsequent repopulation and regeneration of lymphoid organs, is probably merely an acceleration of the normal lymphocyte destruction and lymphoid organ repopulation occurring continuously throughout normal life. Thus it is known that although lymph node small lymphocytes have a long life span, these cells are regularly replaced, and further, that the primitive lymphoid cells in the lymph nodes and spleen are constantly being replaced by blood-borne cells, probably of bone marrow origin.

On this basis it seemed possible to us that adult thymectomy alone should lead to the development of demonstrable immunological defects provided only that sufficient time was allowed to elapse before tests were made. We have tested the haemagglutinin response of C57Bl and (AKR×C57Bl)F_1 mice, thymectomised at 6 weeks of age, to sheep red cells, giving the challenge inoculum at varying intervals after thymectomy. Mice tested immediately after thymectomy produced haemagglutinin titres which were identical with titres in sham operated mice. Mice, challenged for the first time 11 months after operation, produced titres which were significantly lower than in control mice (Fig. 31). The difference seemed most evident on day 5 after challegehe—the time of peak production of 19S antibody. In mice thymectomised 18

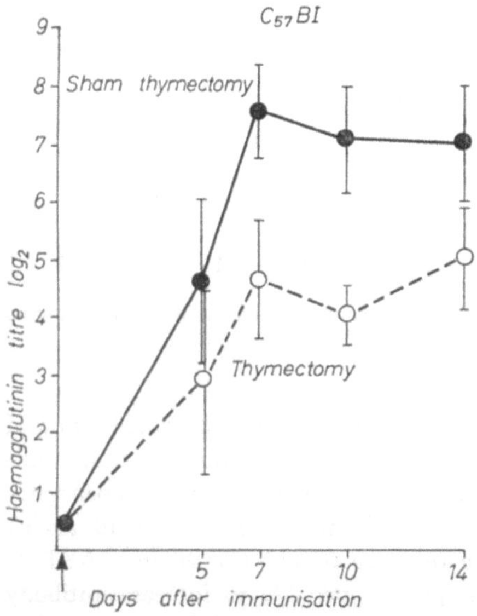

Fig. 31

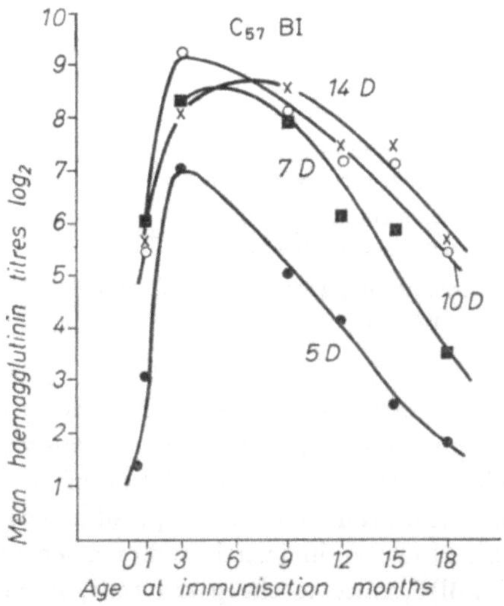

Fig. 32

Fig. 31. Reduced haemagglutinin response to primary immunisation with sheep red cells in C57Bl mice thymectomised at six weeks of age and tested eleven months after operation. Each point is mean value of twelve mice, vertical bars are standard deviations of values

Fig. 32. Decline in the haemagglutinin response to primary immunisation with sheep red cells with increasing age in normal C57Bl mice. Each point is mean value of six mice

months before testing, more than half failed to produce detectable haemagglutinin titres, the remainder producing titres within the rather wide range of titres produced by normal mice of this age (Table 8) (METCALF 1965 b).

It seems clear therefore that the thymus continues to exert an influence over immunological responsiveness throughout life. The effects of thymectomy may be most severe and most rapid in onset when the thymus is removed early in life, but qualitatively similar changes can be observed as a delayed response to thymectomy in adult life.

In some strains of mice at least the ability to produce good haemagglutinin titres in response to primary challenge with sheep red cells declines with advancing age

Table 8. *Primary Haemagglutinin Response of (AKR×C 57 Bl)F_1 Mice to Sheep Red Blood Cells*

Type of mouse	Number of animals	Haemagglutinin titres log 2											
		0	1	2	3	4	5	6	7	8	9	10	11
Normal 2 months old no antigen	14	12		1			1						
Normal 18—20 months old no antigen	18	18											
Thymectomy + antigen 1 week after operation	13									5	7	1	
Sham-thymectomy+antigen 1 week after operation	14									5	6	3	
Thymectomy+antigen 11 months after operation	23			1		3	2	6	10	1			
Sham-thymectomy+antigen 11 months after operation	31							1	13	13	3		1
Thymectomy+antigen 18 months after operation	13	6	1				2			2	2		
Sham-thymectomy+antigen 18 months after operation	48				4	4	4	7	11	12	3	2	1

Immunising Dose — 0.2 ml of 20% sheep R.B.C.I.P. Sera titrated on day 10 following immunisation.

(Fig. 32). It seemed possible that thymectomy may merely produce an acceleration of this age dependent decline in responsiveness—a concept which would be compatible with the continuous repopulation of lymphoid tissues throughout life, its dependency on thymus function and the possible deterioration in thymus function with advancing age. However in initial studies made on the response of old C57Bl and (AKR × C57Bl)F_1 mice to sheep red cells, it has not proved possible to increase antibody responses by grafting up to 12 neonatal thymus glands per recipient, even when challenge was delayed 1—3 months after grafting, by which time massive amounts of young thymus tissue had been present for some months in these animals. It now seems likely that the immune deficiencies of aged mice may stem from a number of associated deficiencies, only one of which is thymus deficiency (Metcalf, unpublished data).

Similar delayed effects of adult thymectomy on immunological competence have been observed by Taylor (1965) and by Miller (1965 a). Miller was able to demonstrate that this decline in competence commenced earlier than indicated by our antibody studies by using the more sensitive plaque forming test of Jerne—adult thymectomised mice showing a fall in the maximum plaque forming cell response to sheep red cells as early as 6 months after adult thymectomy.

It is well known that thymectomy performed on mice in adult life does not lead to any shortening of their mean life span and in some cases (e.g. in high leukaemia strain AKR mice) thymectomy may even prolong the mean life span. This would suggest that such mice are able to cope effectively with the ordinary infectious agents, endemic in all conventional animal colonies, for any serious depression of immune defence systems would be followed rapidly by an increased mortality from infections. This type of sequence is well known following irradiation or cortisone administration. It is likely therefore that the decline in immunological competence following adult thymectomy may only apply to some antigens and not to others.

Before leaving the subject of the relation between the thymus and immune responses, mention should be made of other organs having an analogous role in immune responses.

The bursa of Fabricius in chickens seems to share with the chicken thymus some of the immunological functions carried out by the mammalian thymus. Thus the bursa appears to control the production of circulating antibodies and delayed hypersensitivity reactions in chickens whereas the thymus is concerned with homograft responses (WARNER and SZENBERG, 1964). Bursectomy in early life in chickens (either surgically or by testosterone treatment) profoundly reduces the capacity of chickens to produce a variety of antibodies (GLICK, CHANG and JAAP, 1956; MUELLER, WOLFE and MEYER, 1960) and probably because of this immunological incapacity, bursectomised chickens die prematurely. Grafts of bursal tissue and saline extracts of bursa (GLICK, 1960) partially restored the immune capacity of bursectomised chickens. As far as the production of circulating antibodies in chickens is concerned, the bursa may have the same relationship to the lymphoid tissues of the chicken as the thymus has to the non thymic lymphoid organs in mammals. Recently JANKOVIC and LESKOWITZ (1965) have reported the restoration of haemagglutinin production to human red cells in bursectomised chickens by the grafting of bursal tissue in millipore diffusion chambers, suggesting that the bursa regulates antibody production by other lymphoid cells in the chicken via a humoral factor similar to the thymic humoral factor operating in mammals.

2. Effect of the Thymus on Immune Tolerance

So far we have discussed active immune responses to antigenic stimulation and the role the thymus plays in these immune responses. However the thymus also appears to be involved in a second type of immunological response to foreign antigens—the phenomenon of tolerance.

The term "tolerance" denotes the failure of the body to develop a humoral or cellular immune response when challenged by a foreign antigen, either in the form of injected antigen or of a challenge graft of foreign tissue or cells. The body develops tolerance to a foreign antigen, rather than developing an immune response, when the immunologically reactive tissues of the body are in an immature state or when they have been reduced to a comparable state by various experimental procedures. This development of tolerance to antigenic material which occurs in the immature animal (e.g., the foetus or the neonatal animal) is believed to be the basis of the animal's ability to discriminate "self" from "non-self" antigenic determinants. The tissue antigens present in the animal in foetal life induce a permanent state of tolerance and in subsequent life these antigens are accepted as "self", all other antigens presented to the animal after the phase of immunological immaturity are then recognised as "non-self" and immune responses are developed against them. It is not only normal tissue antigens which can induce tolerance during immunological immaturity. If infecting viruses are present in the animal at this time, these viruses can also induce a state of tolerance so that in later life the foreign viral antigens also are accepted as self with the result that no immune elimination of the virus occurs and a permanent viraemic state results. At least two viruses and possibly a third are known to infect foetal mice and to induce a tolerant state with subsequent permanent viraemia—the lymphocytic choriomeningitis virus (HOTCHIN, 1962), the Gross leukaemia virus (AXELRAD, 1965) and possibly also the mammary tumour virus of Bittner (MORTON, 1964; MORTON, GOLDMAN and WOOD, 1965).

Two features of tolerance need emphasis—1. Tolerance is specific for the antigen inducing the tolerant state—just as specific as is an active immune response to the same antigen. 2. Tolerance to an antigen will only persist so long as that antigen is present in the body. Tolerance to foreign cells or antigens has been induced experimentally in mice, rats and rabbits by introducing the cells or antigen into the animal in the neonatal period. When the introduced foreign cells either proliferate or persist in the animal (e.g. when lymphoid cells or bone marrow cells are used), tolerance may persist for long periods after a single injection of such cells. However with non-replicating antigenic material e. g. bovine serum albumin or sheep red cells, tolerance can only be maintained if repeated injections of the antigen are carried out. NOSSAL and MITCHELL (1965) have carried out quantitative investigations on the dose of antigen required to induce tolerance and the fate of this antigen, when given in doses large enough to induce a tolerant state. They are of the opinion that a tolerance inducing schedule of injections is one in which sufficient antigen has been given to allow exposure of all the lymphoid cells in the body, and possibly particularly the lymphoid cells in the thymus, to that antigen in *a non-phagocytosed state.*

It has been observed that if regular antigen injections are ceased, the tolerant state breaks down and further, that the speed of breakdown of the tolerant state can be accelerated by whole body irradiation (FEFER and NOSSAL, 1962).

The fundamental nature of the process in the lymphoid tissues responsible for the development of tolerance is still uncertain and is the subject of active investigation. The most likely possibilities are 1. that exposure to an antigen in immaturity leads to elimination of those specific cells capable of responding to the particular antigen used (possibly by a combination of the antigen with the cells in the presence of complement, leading to immune lysis of the cell)—the tolerant state is here conceived of as one in which no cells capable of reacting to that specific antigen are present in the body or, 2. that repeated exposure to an antigen in immaturity leads to a suppression of immune reactivity of the specific cells concerned by antibody adherence to the cell surface, blocking the receptor sites on the cell which normally would combine with antigen to initiate an immune response. If individual cells are capable of responding to more than one antigen, then this blocking action, whether mediated by antigen or antibody, may be selective, allowing the cell to take part in active responses to other antigens. This state might be comparable with the differentiated state of other tissues e.g. where a liver cell presumably has permanently suppressed the genetic information contained in it which might allow it to become a pancreatic cell.

Essentially then the tolerant state is either one in which cells which are capable of reacting with the antigen concerned have been eliminated, or one in which potentially reactive cells are present in the body but are blocked from initiating an immune response—"tolerant cells".

Direct studies have now been made in tolerant rats and mice on the content of antigenically reactive cells still present in these animals. ROWLEY and FITCH (1965) have studied rats tolerant to sheep red cells using the Jerne plaque technique which demonstrates single cells capable of producing 19S antibody to sheep red cells. They found tolerant rats to contain far fewer of these cells in the spleen than normal rats and following challenge antigenic stimulation with sheep red cells no, or minimal, proliferation of these cells occurred unlike the situation in the normal animal. MILLER (personal communication) has made similar studies in mice made tolerant to sheep red cells and has demonstrated the existence of an essentially similar situation. These studies make it evident that a tolerant animal, if not lacking reactive cells, certainly has diminished numbers of reactive cells which do not proliferate following antigenic stimulation. The findings do not really discriminate between the two theories of the nature of the tolerant state—cell elimination versus cell reactivity blockade—but since at least some reactive cells are present, the present data tend to favour a functional blockade concept. It will be noted from the results that there is a striking similarity in the response to foreign red cells between neonatally thymectomised animals and tolerant animals.

CLAMAN and TALMAGE (1963) and CLAMAN and MCDONALD (1964) showed that thymectomy of adult rats made tolerant to bovine serum albumin slowed the breakdown of the tolerant state following cessation of regular bovine serum albumin injections. Conversely, SZENBERG and WARNER (1963) showed that thymus grafts from non tolerant chickens placed in chickens previously made tolerant to foreign chicken tissues were capable of breaking down tolerance in such chickens.

In considering how the thymus might influence the rate at which the tolerant state breaks down following removal of the tolerance inducing antigen, various workers have advanced the same types of hypotheses as were advanced to explain the role of the thymus in active immune responses.

It has been postulated by BURNET (1962) that lymphoid cells with the capacity to respond to various antigens are generated on a random basis in the body (in the absence of the appropriate antigen) by random genetic mutations which probably occur at the time of mitosis in these cells. Thus it is postulated that in tissues with active lymphopoiesis, there is a continuous random generation of cells with new reactivity patterns. Those cells arising which can react with "self" antigens are eliminated and the remainder are available for stimulation by specific foreign antigens, should the animal subsequently become exposed to these antigens. BURNET considers that the thymus is the primary organ in the body (1) generating new cells with new reactivity patterns, or additional cells to replenish existing populations of cells with existing reactivity patterns, and (2) eliminating self-reacting cells.

If the tolerant state is one in which reactive cells have been eliminated, then breakdown in tolerance might be expected once antigen administration was ceased because the thymus would continue to generate cells with new patterns and sooner or later would generate cells capable of responding to the antigen concerned. Thymectomy would remove the sole, or major, organ generating cells with new reactivity patterns and thus would greatly slow or prevent tolerance breakdown. This concept has one unexpected virtue in that it would provide a reason for the puzzling extensive, but apparently purposeless, lymphopoiesis and lymphocyte breakdown occurring in the thymus. This lymphopoiesis would then represent the large scale mitotic activity needed to generate new reactivity patterns by random mutation and the extensive lymphocyte breakdown in the thymus, the elimination of self-reactive clones of cells before they can enter the body and damage host tissues.

As has already been pointed out, it seems rather doubtful whether the thymus exports large numbers of the cells produced in the organ. However it is probable that a very small percentage of such cells (less than 0.5%) does enter the body and it is just conceivable that this cell migration might be extensive enough to fulfil the postulated requirements for cells with new reactivity patterns.

ARGYRIS (1965) has recently reported studies on C3H mice made tolerant to CBA tissues by the neonatal injection of CBA spleen cells. These tolerant mice accepted for prolonged periods skin grafts from CBA mice. Tolerance was broken down following grafting of C3H thymus grafts from normal newborn or adult C3H mice. Thus thymus grafting accelerated the spontaneous loss of tolerance which occurs in such mice with advancing age (ARGYRIS, 1962). However ARGYRIS demonstrated that C3H thymus grafts in millipore diffusion chambers also were successful in breaking down tolerance. Clearly this experiment implicates a thymic humoral factor as being involved, in part at least, in the role of the thymus in breaking immune tolerance. This is a most important finding which is in need of confirmation.

If this observation proves correct, the thymic humoral factor (presumably the same humoral factor as is involved in immune responses) may operate by activating precursor cells to become responsive to stimulation by antigen. In this concept, the bone marrow and possibly other tissues are conceived of as producing cells with the genetic make-up allowing responsiveness to stimulation by various antigens—each cell being capable of responding only to a single antigen or to a very few antigens. These cells remain as a pool of inactive "stem cells" until the appropriate antigen is presented to the cells by the antigen trapping and processing macrophage-reticulum cell system. Then, provided thymic humoral factor activates the cell, (cf. erythropoietin activation of an uncommitted stem cell to commence synthesis of haemoglobin) the cells with the appropriate reactivity patterns respond to the antigen by proliferation, forming clones of lymphoid and plasma cells (Fig. 33). If the tolerant state is one in which reactive cells are eliminated or suppressed, once the blocking antigen is no longer present new cells generated by the bone marrow will break the tolerant state—but only if a necessary supply of thymic humoral factor is present to activate them. Thus thymectomy would delay or prevent the breakdown in tolerance by a removing humoral factor and conversely thymus grafts would accelerate tolerance breakdown by providing additional humoral factor (particularly if the production of thymic humoral factor by the host thymus is disturbed by the high doses of antigen present following the induction of tolerance).

If a thymic humoral factor is involved in the breakdown of tolerance, the finding that irradiation accelerates tolerance breakdown may be explained by two observations reporting increased serum levels of a lymphocyte stimulating factor (? thymic humoral factor) in the sera of irradiated animals. METCALF (1959) reported that the sera from LAF_1 and C57Bl mice subjected to whole body irradiation produced a lymphocytosis in baby mice whereas normal LAF_1 and C57Bl sera from mice of the

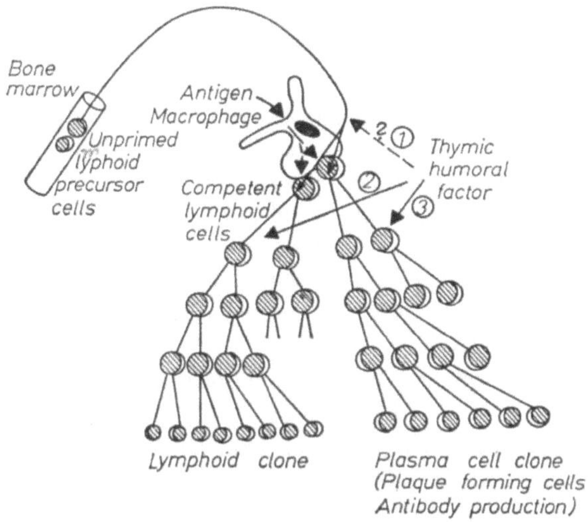

Fig. 33. Schematic representation of role of thymic humoral factor in immune responses. Cells with appropriate reactivity pattern seed in lymphoid tissues (? from bone marrow) and may there be activated by thymic humoral factor to respond to stimulation by macrophage-processed antigen. Thymic humoral factor also stimulates the rate of proliferation of lymphoid and plasma cell clones following antigenic stimulation of activated competent cells

same age were inactive. Similarly ITO and WEINSTEIN (1962) reported that serum from irradiated rats, but not normal serum, when injected into the footpads of test rats increased popliteal lymph node weights and lymph node mitotic activity.

Most studies have indicated that the thymus graft does not *instruct* the lymphoid cells of the thymectomised recipient concerning the antigens against which the restored or activated lymphocytes will react. For example, a neonatally thymectomised strain A mouse, restored to immunological reactivity by a strain B thymus graft will exhibit the immune reactivity of A strain mice, not B strain. Similarly in tolerance, and the breakdown of tolerance, the phenomena observed suggest that the specific reactivity or otherwise resides in the immune tissues themselves and is not dictated by the thymus.

However ISAKOVIC, SMITH and WAKSMAN (1965) have reported that thymus grafts from tolerant animals may confer *specific* tolerance to the thymectomised recipients. Lewis rats aged 5 weeks were thymectomised and at 8 weeks given whole body irradiation. These rats received subsequently thymus grafts from Lewis donors which had been made tolerant to bovine gammaglobulin. Subsequent tests showed that the thymus grafted rats could not be induced to develop delayed sensitisation to bovine gammaglobulin although sensitisation to chicken ovalbumin occurred normally. This observation raises the possibility that the thymus may *confer* the ability to react to specific antigens or to be tolerant to specific antigens. This would need to be via a humoral factor as in the experiment of ISAKOVIC, SMITH and WAKSMAN, the tolerant thymus graft would have been repopulated by non-tolerant host cells and if the graft produced cells for export to the body, they should have been as reactive as the host cells. Alternatively this experiment might be an example of a situation postulated earlier in which the thymus may become damaged by antigen during tolerance induction and may lose its capacity to produce a non-specific humoral factor activating lymphoid cells. Actually this latter situation seems very improbable as a tolerant animal is otherwise healthy and resists infection and responds to other antigens in a normal manner—which would seem to require the presence of adequate levels of thymic humoral factor.

It is apparent that much work needs to be done in analysing completely the nature of the tolerant state and the role of the thymus in this process, but at this stage it seems firmly established that the thymus does accelerate tolerance breakdown and that thymectomy slows spontaneous tolerance breakdown. A thymic humoral factor has been implicated but theoretically production by the thymus of specifically reactive lymphoid cells capable of responding to the antigen could also be involved.

3. Effect of the Thymus in Autoimmune Disease

So far we have discussed two types of immune reactivity—active immune responses and tolerance—both of which are concerned with the response of the body to foreign antigens and both of which occur in normal animals. There remains a third type of immune response, autoimmune response, which is believed not to occur in normal animals and which when it does occur results in disease of the host animal.

An autoimmune response is one in which the animal's own lymphoid tissues respond to stimulation by the animal's own tissue antigens, resulting in the production of lymphoid cells and/or antibodies which react with the normal host tissues causing tissue damage (autoimmune disease).

Various types of autoimmune disease occur in humans and at least one spontaneous type—the autoimmune haemolytic anaemia of New Zealand Black (NZB) mice—has been described in animals.

The fundamental nature of autoimmune disease is still highly controversial. Some workers regard these diseases as resulting from the appearance in the body of abnormal or abnormally reactive lymphoid cells which respond to normal host antigens—an unprovoked assault on normal tissues following on the emergence of abnormal lymphoid cells. Others regard the lymphoid tissues in these disease states as being normal and merely exhibiting their normal function. In this latter concept it is envisaged that the lymphoid tissues are stimulated by foreign antigens or abnormal tissue antigens produced by some triggering damaging influence. In situations where there is cross reactivity between the abnormal antigens and normal tissue antigens, it may be that once stimulated, the host lymphoid tissue response enters a vicious circle by damaging host tissues, thus producing more antigenic material to provide a continuing antigenic stimulus for further lymphoid tissue immune damage of normal host tissues.

In view of the foregoing discussion on the possible role of the thymus in immune responses either by creating lymphoid cells with new reactivity patterns or by producing a humoral factor activating lymphoid cells to respond to antigenic stimulation, it is quite conceivable that the thymus could be involved in autoimmune diseases, regardless of the exact nature of the autoimmune process.

Theoretically, an abnormal thymus might initiate autoimmune disease either by the generation of lymphoid cells with self-reactive patterns (or generate lymphoid cells, which in response to a foreign antigen, could cross react with normal tissues) or alternatively the thymus might produce an abnormal humoral factor or humoral factor in abnormal amounts which might create an abnormally hyperreactive state in the lymphoid tissues allowing them to attack or cross react with host tissues.

In man it has been long known that the thymus is morphologically abnormal in the neuromuscular disease, myasthenia gravis. It is well documented that the thymus is often enlarged in such cases or is actually replaced by a lymphoepithelial tumour. In those cases in which there is not a thymic tumour, it is usual to find in the thymus medulla large lymphoid follicles which contain active germinal centres and phagocytic cells and to find plasma cells in excessive numbers in, and around, the lymphoid follicles. Recently, evidence has been presented that myasthenia gravis is probably an autoimmune disease, in which there is produced an antibody reacting with, and possibly damaging, the A-bands of striated muscle. By the use of immunofluorescent techniques it has been shown that gammaglobulin is bound to the muscle A-bands of affected muscles from patients with myasthenia gravis and an antibody has been demonstrated in the serum of such patients which will combine with normal muscle tissue (Strauss et al., 1960). This tissue apparently shares antigens with thymic epithelial cells and antibody from myasthenic patients also localises in the cytoplasm of thymic epithelial cells (Strauss, 1965).

It was established empirically many years ago that thymectomy often cures or improves myasthenia gravis, particularly in those cases with thymic hypertrophy rather than thymic tumours. This might suggest that the thymus actually initiates the disease process but it could be argued that thymectomy improves the disease state by causing a general depression of immune responsiveness and that the thymus exhibits lymphoid follicles and germinal centres simply because it is one of the target tissues being attacked in the autoimmune process.

The relation of the thymus to other autoimmune diseases of man is less certain. Recently Mackay, Masel and Burnet (1964) have reported that the thymus in patients with systemic lupus erythematosus often exhibits lymphoid follicles and germinal centres similar in morphology to those in myasthenia gravis. Only a few thymectomies have been attempted in this disease and in one or two case reports improvement in the patient's symptoms was noted. However the progress of this disease is notoriously difficult to assess because of spontaneous fluctuations in the severity of the disease and the effect of thymectomy on this disease remains to be firmly established.

Bielschowsky, Helyer and Howie (1957) reported the development of a strain of mice, NZB, in which a high proportion of the mice developed spontaneously an autoimmune haemolytic anaemia. Burnet and Holmes have done much to characterise the nature of this disease. The aetiology of the disease remains uncertain but there is a strong genetic predisposition to the development of the disease (Burnet and Holmes, 1965). Beginning in early middle age, these mice develop a Coombs positive haemolytic anaemia. Their sera also contain an antibody capable of giving an indirect Coombs test with normal mouse red cells. A progressive haemolytic anaemia with severe splenomegaly develops, and most mice of this strain die from this disease when between 12 and 18 months of age. Burnet and Holmes (1964) have shown also that the thymus in these mice, at or before the onset of Coombs positive anaemia, develops medullary lymphoid follicles and germinal centres and excessive numbers of plasma cells.

Conflicting reports have been made on the role of the thymus in this mouse disease. Howie and Helyer (1965) reported that neonatal thymectomy of NZB or F_1 hybrid mice did not prevent the development of the disease. However it was observed that when neonatally thymectomised CBAT6 mice were grafted with NZB thymus grafts, these mice developed a Coombs positive anaemia, autoimmune renal lesions and other signs of autoimmune disease (Howie, 1965). Holmes and Burnet (1965) were unable to confirm the induction of autoimmune disease by grafting NZB thymus glands to F_1 hybrid recipients of various types, and this whole question is in need of further experimental analysis.

It is intriguing that these three spontaneous autoimmune diseases—myasthenia gravis, systemic lupus erythematosus and autoimmune haemolytic anaemia should all exhibit similar lesions of the thymus. It is a little unreasonable to discount all these thymic lesions on the basis of cross reactivity with tissues as widely divergent as muscle, kidney and red cells. However autoimmune diseases are notoriously protean in the divergency of tissues affected and it is still conceivable that the thymus may merely be a target organ commonly affected in this group of diseases.

The role of the thymus in initiating these spontaneous diseases must also remain in doubt at least until the situation in the spontaneous haemolytic anaemia of NZB mice is clarified.

Leaving aside the question of *initiation*, there is now good evidence that the thymus is at least involved in maintaining the disease process via its general influence on the immune reactivity of lymphoid cells and thymectomy may prove to be a promising technique for controlling or reducing the severity of some of these diseases. However thymectomy carries with it the attendant risk of making these patients hypersusceptible to infections and should not be entertained lightly.

Summary

1. The thymus is essential for the development of adequate humoral and cellular immune responses by the body to many foreign antigens. Thymectomy in the neonatal period leads to the rapid development of immunological deficiencies which are frequently so severe as to lead to the death of the animal. Neonatally thymectomised animals fail to respond to many foreign antigens and tolerate foreign tissue and tumour grafts. Immune competence is restored by thymus grafts and by thymus tissue in millipore diffusion chambers.

The thymus influences immune responses by a humoral factor which allows competent lymphoid cells to proliferate, following antigenic stimulation, to form clones of lymphoid cells and clones of plasma cells producing antibody. The thymus possibly may also serve as a production site for immunologically competent cells for use in the other lymphoid organs.

Thymectomy in adult life, particularly if combined with whole body irradiation, leads to similar immune deficiencies.

2. Thymectomy slows the breakdown of tolerance to foreign antigens, following cessation of tolerance-conferring injections of antigen, and thymus grafts accelerate tolerance breakdown.

3. The thymus exhibits lesions (tumours or lymphoid follicles) in a number of autoimmune diseases in man and animals and may be concerned in the genesis of these diseases.

Chapter 7

Trophic and other Functions of the Thymus

From time to time the suggestion has been raised that apart from mediating immune responses, lymphoid cells, may serve as trephocytes in the body—that lymphocytes may either enter cells and inject material into these cells or disintegrate and release breakdown products, providing essential building blocks for the growth or regulation of other cells (LOUTIT, 1962).

Certainly lymphocytes are ubiquitous throughout most tissues of the body and are particularly numerous near cells having high mitotic activity e.g. the epithelium of the bowel or near areas of tissue repair after injury or infection. It has been observed *in vitro*, in mixed cultures of lymphocytes and other cells, (e.g. with thyroid cells or reticulum cells) that lymphocytes continuously enter, leave and re-enter the cytoplasm and nucleus of these other cells, exhibiting high motility whilst inside these cells (HUMBLE, JAYNE and PULVERTAFT, 1956; SHELTON and DALTON, 1959). This phenomenon has been termed "emperipolesis". It has been noted in mixed cultures of tumour cells and lymphocytes that lymphocytes appear to be attracted towards mitotic cells, particularly cells in metaphase, and pass over the cell in an action akin to cutting the umbilical cord of the separating cells (HUMBLE, JAYNE and PULVERTAFT, 1956). It is quite unknown what functions the lymphocytes are performing in these situations but it is difficult to visualise these associations as being concerned with immune responses.

In the case of the thymus, the concept of a trephocytic function for thymic lymphoid cells is particularly attractive for there is little evidence that thymic lymphoid cells enter into any local immune responses whilst in the thymus. Further the autoradiographic data indicate that the thymic lymphocyte population is replaced every 3—4 days and that few whole cells appear to leave the organ.

It could be postulated that thymic lymphopoiesis is a method devised by the body to synthesise cell building blocks of various types. Instead of cells synthesising such building blocks in their cytoplasm and then shedding this cytoplasm, the body may produce large numbers of thymic lymphocytes which are then disrupted to release the required building blocks. This concept at least would begin to rationalise the peculiar behaviour of the thymus in response to stress and infections. If the thymus is conceived of as an organ designed to release immunologically competent lymphocytes, it is strange that in the very situations where such cells should be most needed by the body—in stress and infections—the first response involves a sharp decrease in the size of the thymus due to cortisone induced *dissolution* of thymic lymphocytes. If what the body requires in these situations is not cells, but cell building blocks, then the early dissolution of the large reservoir of cells in the thymus cortex would be an ideal method for mobilising a large quantity of cell building blocks. The nature of such postulated cell building blocks can only be speculated upon, but since thymic lymphocytes are virtually little else but a nucleus with minimal amounts of undifferentiated cytoplasm, nuclear building blocks seem the most likely type involved.

With the use of radioisotopic labelling of cell nuclei it has now been possible to demonstrate the reutilisation of labelled nuclear material derived from lymphocyte nuclei. It was stated earlier that reutilisation of tritiated thymidine (a precursor of DNA) by lymphoid cells in all lymphoid organs is very extensive—in fact so extensive as to limit seriously our ability to interpret cell kinetic studies in these organs (MITCHELL, MCDONALD and NOSSAL, 1963). The most likely source of the labelled material reutilised by lymphocytes in these organs is the breakdown of adjacent, previously labelled, lymphocytes in the same tissues. CRADDOCK et al. (1964) obtained evidence to suggest that in the thymus the primary source of label for reutilisation is the thymic small lymphocyte and that the availability of these cells or their breakdown products influences the amount of injected isotope taken up by the primitive cells of the thymus. It is possible that the availability of breakdown products within organs like the thymus or the lymph node may serve as a rate-limiting influence on the proliferation of primitive cells in these same organs. It frequently has been observed that in germinal centres, the number of pyknotic lymphoid cells parallels the number of mitotic cells in the same germinal centre. In the thymus of a cortisone treated animal it is tempting to speculate that the large amounts of small lymphocyte breakdown material resulting from the initial cortisone-induced lymphocyte dissolution are responsible, in part at least, for determining or making possible the intense regenerative proliferation which subsequently follows in the thymus.

To some extent therefore it seems that lymphoid tissues may well be self-sustaining by the feedback of breakdown products of dying cells which allows new cell formation. Even if the primary purpose of thymic lymphopoiesis is something else, e.g. to generate cells with new antigen receptor patterns, the self-sustaining nature of this lymphopoiesis, due to the trephocytic effects of lymphocyte breakdown products, would be most valuable. The chemical and physical nature of the labelled material reutilised by lymphocytes is not known. Since the reutilised material in tritiated thymidine experiments is reincorporated into the nuclei, the material must at least be nucleoside in nature but it could be much more complex, e.g. nucleoprotein or even nuclear fragments.

Are lymphocyte breakdown products available to other tissues in the body, and if so are they such an important source of building blocks as to influence the function of these tissues? BRYANT (1963) injected tritiated thymidine-labelled lymphoid cells from CBA mice into partially hepatectomised CBA mice and observed labelling in the nuclei of the regenerating liver cells, the intestinal cells and to a lesser degree the lymphoid tissues of the recipients. He felt that the label for reutilisation was derived from dead lymphocytes and was probably in the form of nucleosides or nucleotides.

FICHTELIUS and DIDERHOLM (1961) similarly observed reutilisation of lymphocyte DNA by fibroblasts adjacent to wounds. RIEKE (1962) also observed reutilisation of label from tritiated thymidine labelled lymphocytes injected intraperitoneally into animals with ascites Sarcoma I cells growing in the peritoneal cavity. The spacial intimacy of the passage of label in both experiments suggested that large DNA molecules might be involved in the transfer of label and that they might be incorporated into the recipient cell genome without significant breakdown. CRADDOCK, RYTOMAA and NAKAI (1964) also observed isotopic labelling in the regenerating liver cells of rats at a time after labelling with tritiated thymidine which strongly suggested that lymphocytes were the only likely source of this label.

It can be argued that if lymphocyte breakdown products are available for reutilisation by other cells, then the thymus is probably the most important source of these products since it is the only major lymphoid organ not obviously involved in (or preoccupied with) antigenic responses. Is there any specific evidence linking the thymus with the growth or function of other tissues?

It is an intriguing fact that a striking correlation exists between the total thymic production of lymphocytes and the absolute body weight increase at various ages in mice (METCALF, 1964 a) (Fig. 34). The significance of this correlation is unknown

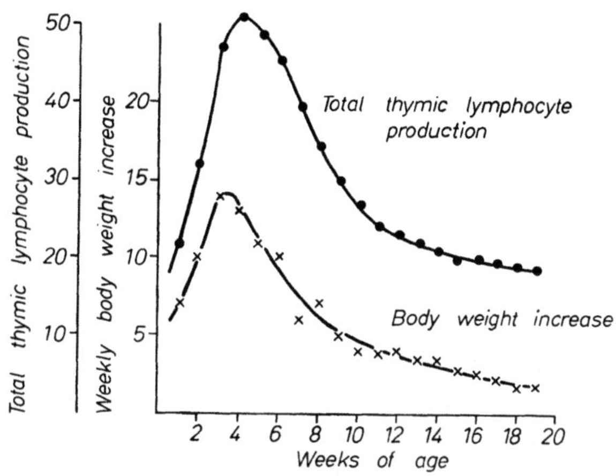

Fig. 34. Correlation between total thymic lymphocyte production (thymus weight in mgm × mean mitoses per 100 thymic lymphocytes) and weekly body weight increase in Gm

but it is at least compatible with the suggestion that the availability of thymic lymphocytes or their breakdown products could be a rate limiting factor in general tissue growth.

It has already been described how animals thymectomised at birth exhibit a reduced rate of growth and even lose weight before death finally occurs. At first this seemed strong evidence implicating the thymus in the regulation of general body growth. However it is now known that neonatally thymectomised animals become hypersusceptible to infections and that this is the probable cause of the ill health and death observed in these animals. In confirmation of this both MCINTIRE, SELL and MILLER (1964) and WILSON, SJODIN and BEALMAR (1964) have reported that neonatally thymectomised germfree mice exhibit normal body growth. Thus the weight loss in conventional neonatally thymectomised mice seems probably to have been the secondary result of infections occurring in these mice. This seems to eliminate the thymus as having any significant direct trophic effect on body growth in the normal animal. However it could be argued that the germfree animal is leading a particularly charmed life and is escaping much of the tissue wear and tear experienced by conventional animals. It is possible that, under natural conditions where the tissues are damaged continuously either by trauma or by infections, the absence of a supply of thymic lymphocyte breakdown products might lead to observable decreases in the rate of tissue growth or regeneration.

Several reports have indicated that thymectomy has an effect on liver regeneration in conventional animals. FACHET et al. (1963) reported that thymectomy in rats, followed by partial hepatectomy, reduced the subsequent mitotic indices of the regenerating liver cells and reduced the volume of these cells. Similarly CRADDOCK, RYTOMAA and NAKAI (1964) reported that adult thymectomy in rats combined with splenectomy reduced the weight attained by the regenerating liver following resection of 40% of the liver, although increased DNA synthesis was observed in the liver cells. Recently MILLER (personal communication) has observed in mice that neonatal thymectomy reduces the mitotic indices of liver cells regenerating following partial hepatectomy.

We were unable to observe any effect of adult thymectomy or of multiple thymus grafting in C3H mice and AKR mice on kidney hypertrophy following unilateral nephrectomy (METCALF, 1964 a).

Alternative tissues which may show the effect of a reduction in the supply of trephocytic lymphocyte products are those in which continuous rapid cell proliferation is occurring e.g. the haemopoietic tissues and the intestinal mucosa. Certainly, neonatal thymectomy leads to the development of anaemia in mice but as previously indicated this is probably the secondary result of infections. We have confirmed that neonatal thymectomy in C3H and non inbred Hall Institute strain mice leads to anaemia, but anaemia only occurred subsequent to the development of obvious ill health in the animals. In such mice haemoglobin and haematocrit levels were subnormal and the red cells exhibited an anisocytosis, poikilocytosis and increased osmotic fragility. These findings are consistent with a simple iron deficiency anaemia secondary to infection. In some mice, activation of latent Eperythrozoon coccoides infections was noted secondary to neonatal thymectomy, and in these mice an active haemolytic anaemia was observed. Thymectomy of adult mice or multiple thymus grafting of adult mice had no effect on haemoglobin and haematocrit levels or on reticulocyte levels and red cell osmotic fragility, either in unstimulated or in repeatedly bled mice (METCALF, 1964 a).

From time to time, suggestions have been made that lymphocytes or thymic lymphocytes may have trephocytic effects, not by cell breakdown, but by actually transforming into other cell types and thus forming a vital source of such cells. The most frequently suggested transformation is that of small lymphocyte to erythroid cell. Thus small lymphocytes have been postulated by YOFFEY (1957) to be the precursor cells of the erythroblasts in the bone marrow. There may be a germ of truth in this latter proposal since it is now known that the primitive cells in spleen and lymph nodes are replaced by new cells carried in the blood and that the probable morphological appearance of these replacement cells is that of the "small lymphocyte". However as indicated earlier it is likely that a marked heterogeneity exists in the cells having the morphology of the small lymphocyte—some actually being erythroid and myeloid precursor cells whilst others are lymphoid precursor cells and others are true small lymphocytes—most of which are already genetically committed to react with particular antigenic patterns. In the specific context of the thymic lymphoid cells, there is no evidence from cell injection studies in lethally irradiated animals that thymic lymphocytes can give rise to erythroid or myeloid cells, only lymphoid cells (Ford and Micklem, 1963). Similarly Harris and Ford (1964) found no evidence of mitotic cells of thymus graft origin in the bone marrows of neonatally thymectomised mice carrying thymus grafts. Thus thymic small lymphocytes may represent a pure population of true *lymphoid* cells containing only precursors of lymphoid cells and bona fide small lymphocytes—antigenically committed or otherwise. Certainly in the studies referred to above no obvious effects of adult or neonatal thymectomy were observed on red cell formation in mice of various strains. Miller et al. (1965) have reported that neonatal thymectomy in the opossum was followed by maturation arrest of erythropoietic cells and the abnormal persistence of these cells in the spleen and lymph nodes of the developing opossum, but it is uncertain what relation these findings have to possible trophic or regulatory functions of the thymus on erythropoiesis.

Despite the lack of strong experimental evidence supporting the concept that thymic lymphoid cells are concerned with erythropoiesis, one intriguing association remains well documented between the thymus and red cell formation. In man, a condition exists in which there is aplasia of the erythroid tissues leading to severe anaemia. This condition has been reported repeatedly as being associated with an epithelial cell tumour of the thymus (Fisher, 1964). Indeed it may be that pure red cell aplasia is invariably accompanied by this thymic tumour. In several cases at least, cure of the red cell aplasia was achieved by resection of the thymic tumour. The mechanisms involved here are unknown. Possibly there are large species differences in the relation between the thymus and erythropoiesis, and the rat and mouse may not be suitable animals in which to demonstrate this relationship. The thymic tumour, by replacing normal thymic tissue, may have created a state equivalent to thymectomy, however thymectomy in humans with myasthenia gravis has not been reported as leading to anaemia. Alternatively, the tumour cells themselves may produce some factor having a toxic effect on the erythroid tissues.

It has frequently been suggested that blood monocytes and tissue macrophages are derived from small lymphocytes and some direct observations have been made to indicate that cells with the morphology of small lymphocytes can transform to phagocytic cells (Rebuck et al., 1964). However the recent isotopic data of Volkman and Gowans (1965; 1965 a) from parabiotic animals and cell injection studies make it likely that most normal blood monocytes and tissue macrophages are derived from cells in the bone marrow. Murray and Woods (1964) have claimed to have observed the appearance in the guinea pig of labelled macrophages following the local injection of tritiated thymidine into the thymus but Nossal (1964) in similar studies was unable to observe any similar transformation. In our laboratory neither thymectomy nor multiple thymus grafting affected either blood monocyte levels or the characteristic pattern of appearance of newly formed monocytes following labelling with tritiated thymidine. It seems unlikely therefore that thymic lymphoid cells are a significant source of precursor cells for body monocytes and macrophages.

So far we have discussed possible trephocytic functions of the thymus in relation to the production of lymphocytes which may transform into other cell types or whose breakdown products may be available for reutilisation by the tissues. Before concluding the discussion of this aspect of thymus function, some comment needs to be made on the possibility that the thymus can influence other tissues by other means, e.g. by endocrine interactions.

The embryological origin of the thymus is similar to that of the thyroid and since some at least of the thymic cells are known to produce a humoral (hormonal) factor, is it possible that this humoral factor enters into feedback relationships with other endocrine organs or is it possible even that the thymus produces multiple humoral factors as does the pituitary or the adrenal?

The effects of endocrine organ resection are probably most readily observed when the organs are resected in the neonatal period. For example gonadectomy of neonatal CE strain mice leads to the development of adrenal cortex carcinomata whereas gonadectomy in adult CE mice is without any similar dramatic effect (Woolley and Little, 1945). On this basis, neonatal thymectomy may be the most suitable technique for investigating the possible existence of endocrine interrelationships between the thymus and other endocrine organs. Law et al. (1964 a) reported that neonatal thymectomy in mice was followed by changes in various endocrine organs. In neonatally thymectomised mice the cells of the anterior pituitary exhibited a reduction in nuclear and cytoplasmic volume in comparison with control mice. Following neonatal thymectomy, the thyroid gland was observed to be atrophic and the epithelial cells of the follicles were flattened and contained less colloid than normal thyroid cells. The incidence of follicles with foamy colloid was also increased in thyroids from neonatally thymectomised mice. In male mice following neonatal thymectomy, the secondary sex characteristics of the male submaxillary gland and kidney failed to develop and spermatogenesis was often incomplete. These are intriguing observations which clearly need further investigation but some caution needs to be exercised in the interpretation of some of the changes as they may be merely secondary effects of the general ill health of these animals. Studies on neonatally thymectomised germfree animals are urgently needed to settle these questions.

Clearly this whole subject of possible endocrine functions of thymic cells and the interrelationships between the thymus and other endocrine organs is in need of further development. Having taken so long to demonstrate a humoral factor produced by the thymus having an action on lymphoid tissues, we should not blind ourselves to the possibility that the thymus, like the pituitary, may produce more than one humoral factor of importance for the body.

Summary

There is some evidence that lymphocytes and thymic lymphocytes provide breakdown products which can be incorporated by other cells in the body. It is not known whether or not these cell breakdown products serve merely as cell building blocks or exert specific regulatory effects on the cells taking them up. Thymectomy appears to reduce the rate of liver regeneration and thymic lymphocyte production correlates with general body growth. Thymic tumours in man are associated with a pure red cell aplasia but experimental studies have tended to discount any special link between the thymus and erythropoiesis or other types of haemopoiesis (other than lymphopoiesis). The thymus may exert an influence on the pituitary, thyroid and gonads but this question needs much more investigation.

Chapter 8

The Thymus and Lymphoid Leukaemia

In the mouse and rat, the thymus is of critical importance in determining susceptibility to lymphoid leukaemia. In fact the studies on this relationship by McENDY, BOON and FURTH (1944) provided the first definitive evidence that the thymus has any functional activity at all in the body. Although the role of the thymus in lymphoid leukaemia development is still not fully understood much has been learned of the basic mechanisms involved.

In some mice lymphoid leukaemia presents as a generalised involvement of all lymphoid tissues with no special predilection for involving any particular organ. However in most mouse strains the thymus appears to be the organ in which the first leukaemic lymphocytes (lymphoma cells) appear (FURTH and BOON, 1945) and the thymus is the most severely affected organ. In AKR mice, in which the incidence of spontaneous lymphoid leukaemia exceeds 90%, the thymic tissues become infiltrated and replaced by a rapidly expanding population of neoplastic lymphoid cells, and a massive thymic lymphoma forms which occupies up to half the chest cavity. Subsequent to thymic lymphoma development, lymphoma tissue accumulates in, and enlarges, other lymphoid organs and ultimately many non-lymphoid organs are infiltrated—particularly the liver and kidney (Figs. 35, 36). Most AKR mice with lymphoid leukaemia have an aleukaemic blood picture with normal or sub normal numbers of lymphoid cells in the blood. However leukaemic cells may usually be seen in the blood despite the small total number of cells and transplantation tests have revealed the presence of lymphoma cells in the blood of all leukaemic mice tested.

Selective inbreeding has been used to increase the incidence of lymphoid leukaemia in mice and this has led to the development of so-called "high leukaemia strains", e.g. the AKR and C58, in which the incidence of leukaemia exceeds 90%. In other strains leukaemia incidence can be increased by whole body irradiation (KAPLAN, 1947), by chemical carcinogens, such as methycholanthrene or urethan (LAW and MILLER, 1950 a), by oestrogens (GARDNER, DOUGHERTY and WILLIAMS, 1944) and by adrenalectomy and gonadectomy (LAW, 1947).

Conversely, the incidence of lymphoid leukaemia can be decreased by cross mating with low leukaemia strains, foster nursing on low leukaemia strain mice (LAW, 1954), underfeeding (SAXTON, BOON and FURTH, 1944) and cortisone (UPTON and FURTH, 1954) or testosterone administration (MURPHY, 1944).

It has now been shown that leukaemia-inducing viruses can be isolated from many mice with leukaemia. These viruses appear to belong to one or other of two families of related viruses, of which the Gross virus (isolated from AKR mice) causing lymphoid leukaemia and the Friend virus (isolated from Swiss mice) causing erythroleukaemia and reticulum cell sarcoma are the prototypes (GROSS, 1964). A full discussion of leukaemia-inducing viruses in outside the scope of this monograph but certain characteristics of the lymphoid leukaemia-inducing viruses need a brief description to establish a basis for the discussion of the role of the thymus in the development of this disease.

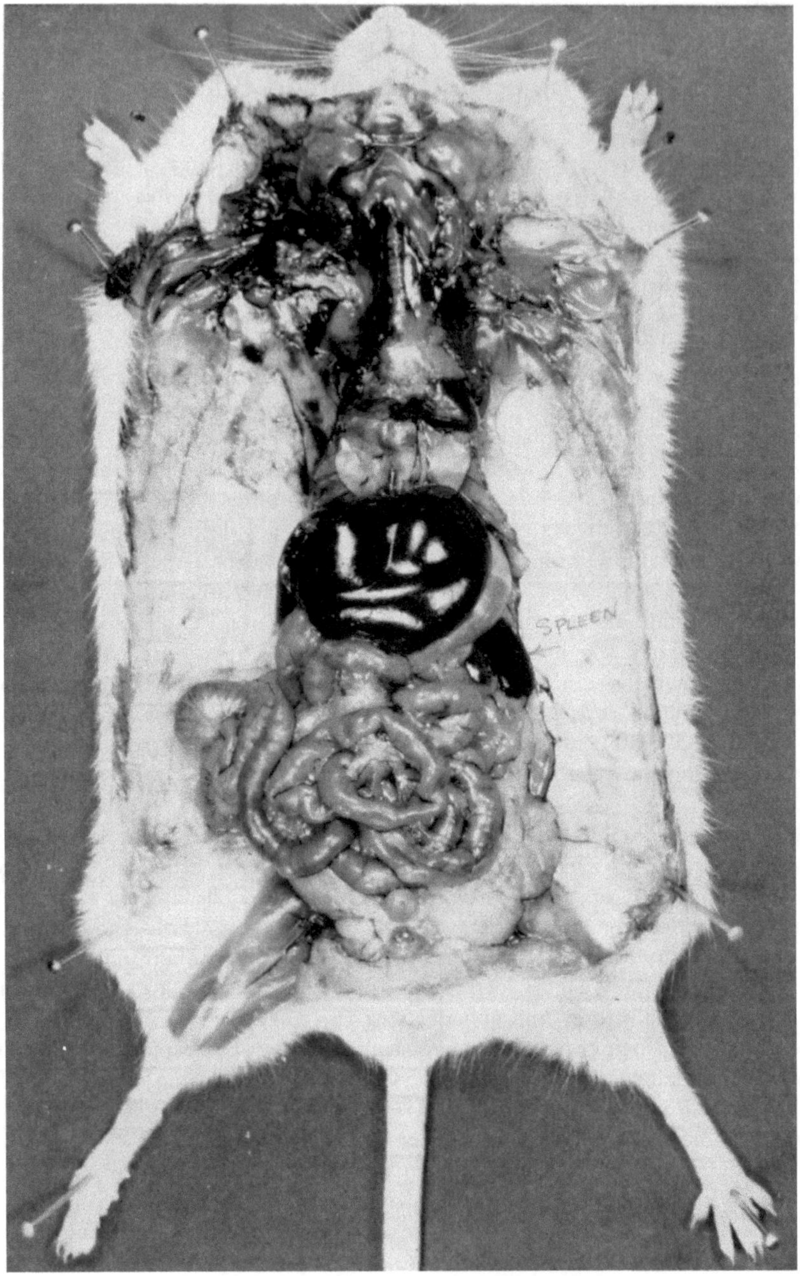

Fig. 35. Normal two months old AKR mouse

The lymphoid leukaemia-inducing viruses do not appear to be infectious in the classical sense. In natural infections by these viruses, the virus passes from one mouse to another by vertical transmission. Thus in AKR mice, which carry a natural infec-

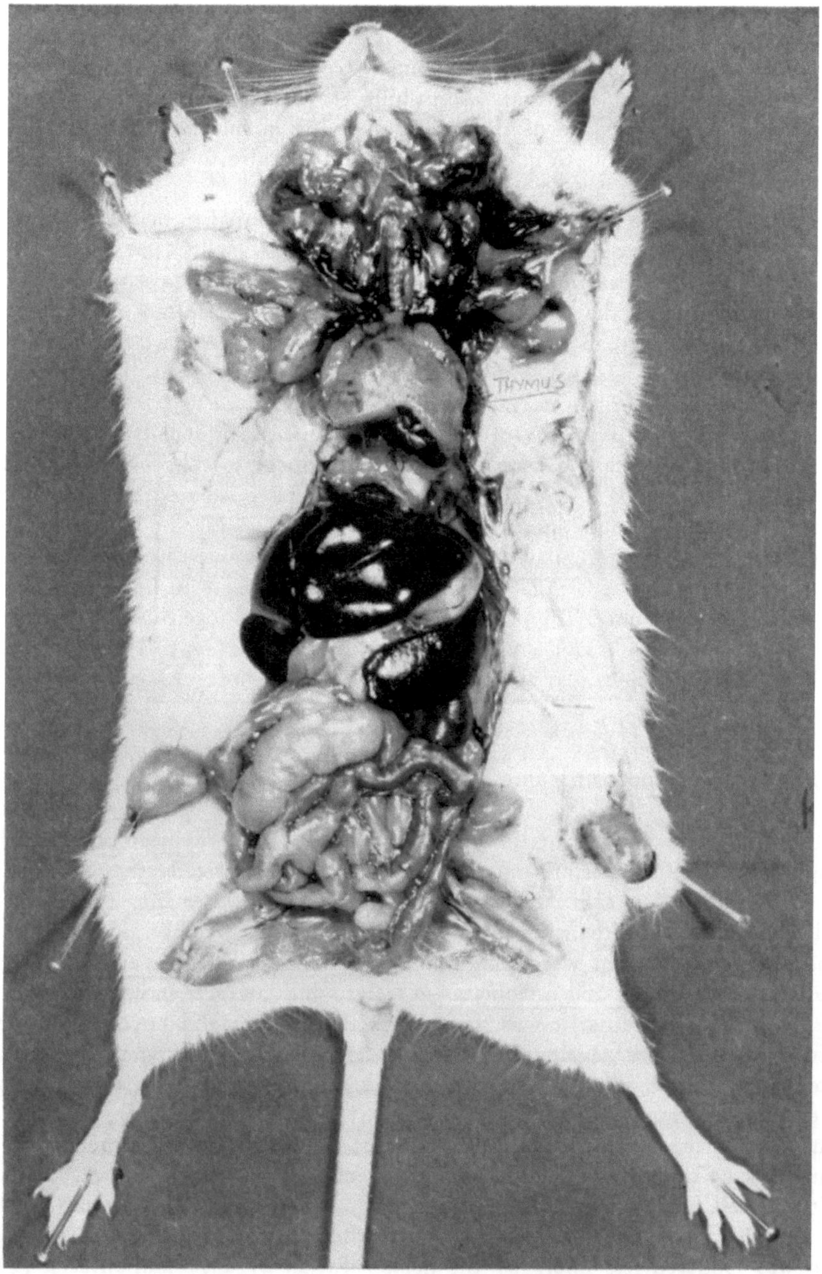

Fig. 36. Eight months old AKR mouse with thymic and generalised lymphoid leukaemia. Note large thymic lymphoma and gross enlargement of subcutaneous and mesenteric lymph nodes

tion by the Gross virus, the virus apparently enters the offspring via the ovum and sperm, and possibly also via the placenta and milk (see review by MILLER, 1961 b). With the Moloney virus, transmission appears to be almost entirely via the milk (LAW,

1962). In natural infections there is a characteristically long latent period between infection and the development of lymphoid leukaemia. This latent period may be a major fraction of the life span of the animal. Coupled with the vertical mode of virus transmission is the fact that susceptibility to infection is highest in the very young. Experimental passage of these viruses results in increased virulence of the viruses which are then able to infect older animals and also to induce a higher incidence of leukaemia with a reduced latent period.

In the AKR mouse, infectious virus may be demonstrated in many tissues of the embryo or the adult mouse in the preleukaemic period (GROSS, 1951). This virus is difficult to visualise in sections examined with the electron microscope but is most readily seen in the megakaryocytes of the bone marrow and spleen (DALTON et al., 1961). However, in animals (rats) infected experimentally with passaged Gross virus, it has been found by OKANO, KUNII and FURTH (1963) that the thymus contains more virus than other organs during the preleukaemic period.

It is now believed that many of the procedures used to induce lymphoid leukaemia in mice may operate by activating latent infections by leukaemia viruses. Thus LIEBERMAN and KAPLAN (1959) and KAPLAN (1965) have isolated repeatedly, from lymphoid leukaemic tissues induced in C57Bl mice by whole body irradiation, a leukaemia-inducing virus similar in character to the Gross virus isolated from AKR leukaemic mice, and GROSS (1959) has isolated what appears to be a similar virus from irradiated C3H mice. The position with chemical carcinogen-induced leukaemia is less certain but there have been initial reports of the isolation of leukaemia-inducing viruses from such mice (TOTH, 1963; GRAFFI, 1965).

1. Effect of Thymectomy and Thymus Grafts on Leukaemia Development

MCENDY, BOON and FURTH in 1944 demonstrated that thymectomy performed on high leukaemia AKR strain mice in early adult life drastically reduced the incidence of lymphoid leukaemia developing in these mice in later life. The thymectomised mice lived longer than the sham operated mice and, possibly as a consequence of their longer life span, were found to develop late in life myeloid leukaemia, reticulum cell sarcomata and osteomata—diseases which are rare in unoperated AKR mice. In subsequent studies it was shown that thymectomy did not affect the proliferative rates of fully developed lymphoma cells. Thus thymectomised mice transplanted with lymphoma cells died as rapidly with transplanted leukaemia as transplanted sham operated mice (FURTH and BOON, 1945).

In AKR mice, as described above, the first neoplastic cells appear within the thymus and the thymus is the most severely affected organ in the disease. Because of this it was felt initially that thymectomy may have prevented leukaemia development simply by removing the tissue most susceptible to neoplastic change. This explanation was rendered less likely by the demonstration by LAW and MILLER (1950) that thymectomy also reduced the incidence of lymphoid leukaemia in C58 mice—one of the strains of mice in which the thymus is not involved regularly in the leukaemic process. It was shown soon after that adult thymectomy also prevented the induction of lymphoid leukaemia by chemical carcinogens (LAW and MILLER, 1950 a) and by whole body irradiation (KAPLAN, 1950).

A great deal of work has been done on the induction of lymphoid leukaemia in mice by whole body irradiation and on the role the thymus plays in this process (see review by KAPLAN, 1954). Thus whole body irradiation, given in fractionated doses to young adult mice induces a high incidence of lymphoid leukaemia. Shielding of part of the body or the injection of normal bone marrow or spleen cells after irradiation reduces the incidence of leukaemia. Thymectomy is most effective in preventing the development of lymphoid leukaemia when performed before, or immediately after, exposure to irradiation but KAPLAN also showed that thymectomy postponed until almost the end of the preleukaemic period was still relatively effective in reducing lymphoid leukaemia incidence, even when the resected thymus showed evidence of lymphoma cells.

The frequency of subsequent lymphoid leukaemia development following irradiation has been correlated with abnormal thymic regeneration—the thymic cells passing through a long period of maturation arrest during the regenerative phase in those animals which will subsequently develop leukaemia. Partial body shielding or the injection of normal bone marrow cells restores a normal pattern of thymic regeneration and reduces the subsequent incidence of lymphoid leukaemia (KAPLAN, BROWN and PAULL, 1953 a). There were some indications that cell free extracts of normal bone marrow might prevent lymphoid leukaemia development in irradiated mice but most experiments indicated the necessity for using viable bone marrow cells for protective effects.

These data on the irradiation induction of lymphoid leukaemia now seem capable of reinterpretation on the basis that irradiation induces lymphoid leukaemia indirectly by activating latent lymphoid leukaemia viruses in the animal. Such viruses have now been isolated repeatedly from irradiation-induced lymphoid leukaemia. If the activation of such viruses depends on a breakdown by the irradiation of some immune process holding the virus in check, then partial body shielding or the injection of healthy bone marrow or spleen cells (in the presence of the thymus) would allow a rapid restoration of immune responses, and this might be expected to keep the lymphoid leukaemia virus in a latent (? suppressed) form. The role of the incomplete or arrested thymic regeneration in the leukaemogenic process is less certain and will be discussed later. Certainly from what is now known of thymus repopulation by bone marrow and spleen cells, it is likely that seeding and proliferation of such cells in the thymus of irradiated animals accounts for the prompt regeneration of the thymus in irradiated animals injected with bone marrow or spleen cells, or in irradiated mice in which autologous seeding occurs from shielded bone marrow cells.

Subsequent to the development of potent preparations of passaged Gross leukaemia virus, it was shown that thymectomy also prevents the viral induction of lymphoid leukaemia (MILLER, 1959; LEVINTHAL, BUFFETT and FURTH, 1959; GROSS, 1959 a). Testing of virus-injected thymectomised mice by MILLER showed that thymectomy does not prevent virus infection and apparently does not prevent the proliferation of leukaemia virus in the infected animal—although this question still remains uncertain in view of the present extreme difficulty in titrating leukaemia viruses (MILLER, 1960 b). Certainly serial thymectomy in twelve successive generations of AKR mice did not reduce their ability to pass on virus to succeeding generations of offspring and did not reduce the effectiveness of the virus in inducing lymphoid leukaemia in sham operated litter mates (MILLER, 1962 c).

Subcutaneous thymus grafts restore the susceptibility to lymphoid leukaemia of thymectomised mice—whether the lymphoid leukaemia is of the spontaneous (Law and Miller, 1950; Miller, 1960 a), virus-induced (Miller, 1960; Levinthal and Buffett, 1961), carcinogen induced (Law and Miller, 1950 a) or irradiation induced type (Kaplan, Brown and Paull, 1953). Usually the thymus graft is the site of development of the first lymphoma cells and the graft is transformed into a massive lymphosarcoma. Although the host organs subsequently may be enlarged by lymphoma cell infiltration, the graft usually remains as the largest mass of lymphoma tissue.

In thymectomised F_1 hybrid mice, made by crossing high and low leukaemia strain mice, it has been shown that susceptibility to lymphoma development is restored by thymus grafts from the high leukaemia strain parent but not by grafts from the low leukaemia strain parent (Law, 1959). Similarly Miller (1960 a) found that C3H thymus grafts in thymectomised C3H mice did not induce lymphoid leukaemia development, but AKR thymus grafts in C3H mice (made tolerant at birth to AKR tissues) did lead to a significant incidence of lymphoid leukaemia, most leukaemias developing in the graft site. Kaplan has shown a similar phenomenon with thymectomised irradiated (C57Bl × C3H)F_1 mice—susceptibility to lymphoid leukaemia being conferred by C57Bl thymus grafts but not by C3H thymus grafts (Kaplan, Hirsch and Brown, 1956). These experiments are reminiscent of earler experiments with lung grafts—genetic susceptibility to urethan-induced lung tumours apparently being resident in the cells of the lung tissue itself.

In the case of thymus grafts however, the situation is more complex for, as discussed earlier, all thymus grafts are chimaeric tissues being composed of donor epithelial and reticulum cells and host lymphoid cells. Since lymphoma cells are neoplastic *lymphoid* cells, lymphomata arising in thymus grafts might be expected always to be derived from host cells. Transplantation tests and chromosome marker studies have in fact confirmed that many such graft lymphomata—although originating in the grafts—are derived from host cells. In the earlier description of the repopulation of normal thymus grafts, evidence was presented that by three to four weeks after grafting 100% of graft lymphoid cells are of host origin. Somewhat surprisingly, the percentage of lymphomata of host cell origin in thymus grafts is not 100%, most of the observed percentages varying from 30—80%.

Law and Potter (1956) showed that thymectomy prevented the induction of lymphoid leukaemia in (C57Bl × A)F_1 mice by whole body irradiation and that thymus grafts from C57Bl donors partially restored the ability of such animals to develop lymphoid leukaemia. However when the genotype of the leukaemic cells was determined by test transplantations in C57Bl and (C57Bl × A)F_1 mice, in only 8 of 12 cases tested were the leukaemic cells demonstrated to have arisen from F_1 host cells. However Law (1952) had earlier found in thymectomised (C3H × AKR)F_1 mice grafted with AKR thymus grafts that all of 6 lymphomata tested which arose in the graft site were derived from host F_1 hybrid cells.

Similar evidence was obtained by Barnes et al. (1959) who studied the leukaemias arising in (C57Bl × T6)F_1 mice thymectomised, irradiated and grafted with C57Bl thymus grafts. On the basis of transplantation and chromosome analysis of 15 of these lymphomata, only 7 were shown to have originated from F_1 host cells (and to contain T6 marker chromosomes).

Similarly, MILLER (1961 a) found in (AKR × T6)F_1 mice thymectomised and grafted with AKR thymus grafts that 5 of 6 lymphomata arising in the thymus grafts contained T6 marker chromosomes in their dividing cells indicating an origin of the neoplastic cells from host cells, although neoplasia developed in the thymus graft itself.

LEVINTHAL and BUFFETT (1961) reported that in virus-infected thymectomised (AKR × C3H)F_1 mice developing lymphoid leukaemia after being grafted with parental strain thymus grafts, 8 of 13 lymphomata in thymus grafts were of F_1 host origin.

KAPLAN (1965) has recently made a more critical analysis of the origin of lymphoma cells arising in thymus grafts. In his system, passaged leukaemia virus was injected directly into parental thymus grafts at various intervals after placing the grafts under the kidney capsule of thymectomised F_1 hybrid recipients. In this system a very high incidence of graft lymphomata resulted with a very short latent period (possibly only days in length). Test transplantations of lymphomata arising in such grafts revealed that the ratio of lymphomata of donor origin to those of host cell origin followed exactly the pattern of host replacement of donor mitotic lymphoid cells reported for kidney subcapsular thymus grafts by METCALF, WAKONIG-VAARTAJA and BRADLEY (1965). Thus at day 20 after grafting, when 50% of mitotic cells in such grafts are of host origin, so 50% of lymphomata were derived from host cells and after day 35 following grafting, only host type lymphomata were obtained.

These recent results suggest that it should only be possible to obtain graft lymphomata of donor origin for as long as donor mitotic lymphoid cells persist in the grafts. This makes it somewhat difficult to explain the donor origin of graft lymphomata arising in the earlier experiments of a number of investigators, in which subcutaneous grafts were used (which are rapidly repopulated by host cells) and in which relatively long latent periods (months) elapsed before lymphomata occurred in the grafts.

Several possibilities could account for this latter type of observation. It was suggested by ARNESEN (1958 a) that some so-called "lymphomata" may not be neoplasms of lymphoid cells but be morphologically similar epithelial neoplasms derived from the thymic epithelial cells. If this is so, then it would explain the donor origin of some graft lymphomata, for the epithelial cells of thymic grafts remain donor in type. Alternatively the graft epithelial cells may recommence the formation of lymphoid cells at some stage in the preleukaemic period in a manner similar to the proposed epithelial cell generation of lymphocytes in the embryonic thymus (AUERBACH, 1961). In support of this possibility we have observed higher mitotic activity in the epithelial cells of the preleukaemic AKR thymus than in the thymus of other strains of mice at a similar age. However it is more likely that the donor origin of some graft lymphomata may be due to donor cell migration from the graft to the host, and then from the host back to the thymus graft. It is known that some graft lymphoid cells escape from the thymus grafts (probably in the immediate post-grafting period) and seed and proliferate in host lymphoid organs (LEUCHARS, CROSS and DAVIES, 1964). If some of these cells subsequently re-migrated to the thymus graft they might well become neoplastic if these donor-strain cells were more susceptible to neoplastic change than those of the host. In this regard it has been shown that when AKR spleen cells are injected into (AKR × C3H)F_1 mice, some at least of the cells can seed in the thymus, and at a subsequent time, give rise to thymic lymphomata derived from the AKR cells (METCALF, 1963 a).

While for the present the donor origin of some thymus graft lymphomata remains an unsolved problem, the fact remains that most lymphomata arising in thymus grafts are derived from host cells which have become neoplastic in the environment of the thymus graft. Since thymus grafts from other strains of mice in the same type of host animal are unable to induce lymphoid leukaemia development, this observation indicates that the simple mechanistic explanation of the effect of thymectomy in preventing lymphoid leukaemia (by the removal of susceptible cells) is either not correct or not the whole explanation. Clearly part of the role of the thymus in leukaemogenesis is an indirect one—the thymus of certain strains (but not others) appears able to induce the host cells repopulating the thymus graft to become neoplastic.

What are the differences between high leukaemia strain thymus glands (which can confer susceptibility to lymphoid leukaemia) and low leukaemia strain thymus glands (which cannot)? The AKR thymus is larger than that in low leukaemia strain mice and AKR primitive thymic lymphoid cells proliferate slightly more rapidly than those in low leukaemia C3H strain thymus glands. Thymus graft experiments described earlier indicated that the AKR thymic epithelial and reticulum cells exert a more powerful proliferative stimulus than low leukaemia strain C3H thymic cells.

(AKR × C3H)F_1 mice in our laboratory develop a 90% incidence of lymphoid leukaemia as do the parental strain AKR mice. However the F_1 hybrid mouse develops leukaemia more slowly (mean latent period to leukaemia development 52 weeks, versus mean latent period to leukaemia development in AKR mice of 32 weeks). When AKR thymus grafts were placed in (AKR × C3H)F_1 mice, no acceleration of leukaemia development was observed and although some of the grafts developed primary lymphomata, not as many did so as might have been anticipated (METCALF, 1964 b). Since F_1 hybrid cells repopulate the AKR grafts, it appears as if the intrinsic suceptibility to neoplasia development of these F_1 cells is what determines the length of the latent period and not the strength of the thymic influence (which is presumably greater in the AKR thymus than in the F_1 thymus).

These data, combined with the earlier results of LAW and KAPLAN, suggest that two distinct components are operating in thymus graft-induced lymphoid leukaemia development (a) The strength or nature of the epithelial and reticulum cell influence—AKR being stronger than C3H, and C57Bl being stronger than C3H—which determines whether or not lymphoid leukaemia can occur; and (b) The susceptibility of the thymic lymphoid cells to this leukaemogenic influence—AKR cells being more susceptible than (AKR × C3H)F_1—which determines the length of the latent period to leukaemia development and possibly the final incidence of lymphoid leukaemia.

Is the difference between the epithelial and reticulum cell influence of the AKR and the C3H thymus simply a quantitative one? We have investigated this by observing the effects on the incidence of leukaemia of multiple C3H thymus grafts in C3H mice. Up to 10 C3H grafts per recipient failed to induce leukaemia development in these recipients (METCALF, WIADROWSKI and BRADLEY, 1965). If there is merely a quantitative difference in function between the AKR and C3H thymus then apparently this difference is greater than a tenfold one. The same experiment makes it seem unlikely that thymus tissue confers susceptibility to leukaemia simply by providing a large number of rapidly dividing lymphoid cells, which on a random mutation basis, are prone to neoplasia, for multiple thymus grafted animals have a larger mass of thymus tissue than does the AKR animal.

Is the leukaemogenic influence of an AKR thymus a positive influence or is the AKR thymus unable to perform some function (for example, surveillance function) which a C3H thymus can perform? Working on the assumption that the thymus in (AKR × C3H)F_1 mice is unable to perform a vital function, normally suppressing the emergence of leukaemic cells, we have attempted to correct this hypothetical defect by grafting F_1 mice each with two low leukaemia strain C3H thymus grafts early in life. This procedure had no inhibitory influence on the incidence of lymphoid leukaemia or on the latent interval to leukaemia development (METCALF, WIADROWSKI and BRADLEY, 1965). In parallel experiments, C3H whole spleen grafting with or without splenectomy of the host also failed to inhibit lymphoid leukaemia development.

The recent overwhelming evidence implicating leukaemia viruses at the initiating agents for lymphoid leukaemia develpoment makes it necessary to consider how this fact can be related to the essential role played by the thymus in the disease process.

Various suggestions have been made to account for the essential role of the thymus in this disease:

1. Leukaemia virus may only reach critical concentrations in the thymus.

2. Infected lymphoid cells may only develop neoplastic change when the virus is able to pass freely from one infected primitive lymphoid cell to another—that is where aggregates of primitive lymphoid cells exist (as in the thymus). Alternatively the very rapidly dividing thymic lymphoid cells may sustain a special type of damage following virus infection which leads to neoplastic change.

3. Viral infection of the special thymic epithelial and reticulum cells may be the critical step in leukaemogenesis and neoplastic lymphoid cells may result from a disturbance of the normal regulatory processes exerted by thymic epithelial and reticulum cells on lymphoid cells.

4. Thymic lymphoid cells may be a special type of lymphoid cell, specially prone to neoplastic change following viral infection.

5. The thymus may offer a safe haven for the survival and proliferation of abnormal preleukaemic cells.

These suggestions will now be discussed along with the evidence on which they are based.

1. In virus infections, the outcome of the virus infection of host cells can depend on the multiplicity of infectivity—that is, the number of virus particles available to infect each host cell. It is conceivable that with tumour viruses, small numbers of virus particles in relation to the population of susceptible cells may lead to the development of a carrier state, whereas high levels of virus may lead to a special type of virus-host cell relationship in which the host cells becomes neoplastic. As a corollary to this proposition, the preleukaemic period may represent the time required for virus titres to rise sufficiently to be able to induce a neoplastic outcome of the virus—host interrelationship. It may be for this reason in AKR mice that the injection of additional virus reduces the length of the latent period to leukaemia

development—the phenomenon of superinfection (RUDALI, DUPLAN and LATARJET, 1956; LATARJET, 1959).

Many workers feel that the thymus is necessary for the development of lymphoid leukaemia because it may be only in the thymus that titres of the leukaemia virus reach critical levels necessary before infected host cells undergo neoplastic change rather than simply enter a carrier state. In support of this concept is the evidence of OKANO, KUNII and FURTH (1963) that, in the preleukaemic period, virus was present in greatest amounts in the thymus, in rats infected with passaged Gross virus. If this observation is correct, there would appear to be some difference between the situation in experimentally versus naturally infected animals, for in the naturally infected state as judged from AKR mice, virus particles are scanty in the preleukaemic thymus and those which are identifiable seem usually to be in epithelial or reticulum cells.

KAPLAN and HARAN-GHERA have carried out some interesting studies on the effect of direct injection of leukaemia virus into thymus grafts. They confirmed the earlier observations of LAW, BRADLEY and ROSE (1963) that whereas thymus grafts in the subcutaneous tissues restored susceptibility to lymphoid leukaemia in thymectomised irradiated C57Bl mice, similar grafts under the kidney capsule did not. However HARAN-GHERA and KAPLAN (1964) found that if virus was injected directly into the thymus graft under the kidney capsule a high incidence of graft and generalised lymphomata resulted. They postulated that for some reason in the injected animals, critical levels of virus cannot be built up in thymus grafts under the kidney capsule. This may be true, but it is difficult to envisage a mechanism preventing virus penetration and proliferation in graft tissue under the kidney capsule. Thymus graft epithelial and reticulum cells survive and grow under the kidney capsule much better than in the subcutaneous tissues but lymphoid repopulation by host cells occurs as with subcutaneous grafts. If host lymphoid *cells* can enter thymus grafts, virus from the irradiated host animal also should have little difficulty in entering the graft.

2. KAPLAN (1961) has suggested that it is only in situations where there is a high cell density of primitive lymphoid cells that leukaemia virus/host cell interaction is of a type leading to leukaemia development. Thus the thymus is postulated to be essential because it is the only organ containing a sufficiently high concentration of such primitive cells. In support of this thesis is the fact that neonatal animals are the most susceptible to infection by leukaemia viruses and in these animals a high percentage of primitive cells is present in the thymus, often as a distinct subcapsular layer (AXELRAD and VAN DER GAAG, 1962). Further, aggregates of primitive lymphoid cells occur in subcutaneous thymus grafts placed in mice subjected to leukaemogenic doses of whole body irradiation (CARNES and KAPLAN, 1956). In subcutaneous thymus grafts there is a relatively long period during which there is apparent failure of what primitive lymphoid cells are present in the cortex to proliferate and differentiate to form small lymphocytes. This could be a significant factor in determining behaviour differences between the susceptibility of subcutaneous and kidney subcapsular thymus grafts in irradiated hosts to undergo neoplastic change for METCALF, WAKONIG-VAARTAJA and BRADLEY (1965) have shown that this period of arrested lymphocyte differentiation and proliferation is much shorter in thymus grafts under the kidney capsule than in similar subcutaneous grafts. However this concept of the specially susceptible nature of aggregates of primitive lymphoid

cells cannot really account for the essential role of the thymus, as aggregates of such primitive lymphoid cells occur in other sites in the body e.g. the germinal centres in lymphoid deposits in lymph nodes, spleen and Peyer's patches.

It has also been postulated that thymic lymphoid cells may be prone to the development of neoplastic change following infection by leukaemia viruses because of their very rapid rate of multiplication (METCALF, 1962). This suggestion is in line with the observation that factors stimulating lymphoid cell proliferation increase the incidence of lymphoid leukaemia and vice versa (KAPLAN, NAGAREDA and BROWN, 1954). However, recent autoradiographic data from tritiated thymidine labelled mice have made it likely that thymic lymphocyte proliferative rates are not as much in excess of lymph node lymphocyte proliferative rates as was formerly believed (METCALF, 1965) and the small differences involved seem scarcely adequate to account for the large difference in susceptibility to neoplastic change between the two populations.

3. An alternative view of the special role of the thymus in virus induced leukaemogenesis is to postulate that it is viral infection of the epithelial and reticulum cells of the thymus which is the critical event rather than infection of thymic lymphocytes. Certainly in the preleukaemic AKR mouse, virus is most evident in the non lymphoid cells of the thymus (DE HARVEN, 1964) and, even in lymphoma cells themselves, virus is not prominent. Virus infection of the thymic epithelial and reticulum cells may disturb the functional interrelationships between the epithelial and reticulum cells and the lymphocytes, and by so doing, disturb the regulation of lymphocyte proliferation and differentiation (FURTH, 1965). Neoplasia development in the lymphoid cells may be an indirect effect resulting from prolonged functional disturbance of this regulation of the lymphoid cells. The ability of a thymus graft from a high leukaemia strain animal to restore susceptibility to leukaemia development in thymectomised F_1 hybrid mice would then hinge on the viral content of the thymus graft epithelial and reticulum cells. Grafts from low leukaemia strain mice would not confer susceptibility to leukaemia development because their epithelial and reticulum cells are not infected by leukaemia virus.

Since the epithelial, and possibly the reticulum cells, of the thymus are unique to the thymus and occur nowhere else in the body, if infection of these cells is a necessary prerequisite for leukaemogenesis, this unique localisation of these cells to the thymus might account for the essential role played by the thymus in this disease.

4. The possibility cannot be excluded that thymic lymphoid cells are a special cell type—not present elsewhere in the body. Although it is known that thymic lymphoid cells are repopulated by host cells probably originating in the bone marrow, it cannot be assumed that these repopulating cells are identical with the bone marrow cells that repopulate the lymph nodes and spleen and it may also be that these thymus seeding cells undergo further changes in the environment of the thymus which render these cells uniquely susceptible to the leukaemogenic action of the infecting leukaemia virus. The cell injection studies of FORD and MICKLEM (1963) suggest that thymic lymphoid cells do become altered after residence in the thymus. The thymus of irradiated animals was found to be repopulated by cells seeding out from injected bone marrow or spleen cells. However, injection studies on these thymic lymphoid cells demonstrated that, having resided in the thymus, they were no longer capable of repopulating the thymus of other irradiated recipients (HARRIS and FORD, 1964).

Similarly the antigen studies of REIF and ALLEN (1964) suggest that thymic lymphocytes contain a special antigen not present in other lymphoid cells, and this antigenic difference may indicate a different functional state of the thymic lymphoid cells which may be coupled with a high degree of susceptibility to neoplastic change.

5. There is a possibility that the interior of an AKR thymus (or of the thymus from other strains which can confer susceptibility to lymphoid leukaemia) may offer a safe haven for the emergence of leukaemic cells, as this process could continue in the host thymus even when low leukaemia strain thymus grafts are placed in the same animal. In fact there is some evidence that the thymus may provide a suitable environment for the survival of abnormal preleukaemic cells. STICH (1963) and JONEJA and STICH (1963) have shown, in animals exposed to leukaemogenic doses of dimethylbenzanthracene or x-irradiation, that lymphoid cells with chromosome abnormalities may be found initially in many haemopoietic organs, but the number of these cells decreases sharply with time. In the thymus of such animals, the number of abnormal cells increases progressively suggesting that perhaps the interior of the thymus does offer a specially suitable site or safe haven for the emergence, survival and proliferation of preleukaemic and leukaemic cells. Similarly ILBERY et al. (1962) demonstrated that lymphoid cells with abnormal chromosome complement were proliferating in the preleukaemic thymus following whole body irradiation. It is uncertain what mechanisms might allow selective survival of abnormal preleukaemic cells in the thymus. However if these cells contain foreign antigens, as is quite possible, then the absence of local immune responses in the thymus may be of relevance, for antigenic cells located in the thymus might then not be subject to attack by host lymphoid cells.

2. Preleukaemic Changes in the Thymus

In this discussion the term "preleukaemic" needs some amplification. AKR mice are known to be infected with the Gross virus in its native form before birth but they do not commence dying from leukaemia until the age of 6 months (Fig. 37). This

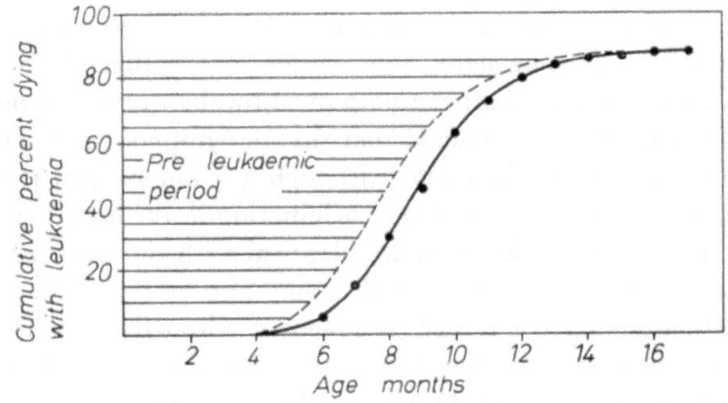

Fig. 37. Figure showing cumulative mortality from lymphoid leukaemia in AKR mice. Broken line represents time of first appearance of leukaemic cells in the thymus and the hatched area the preleukaemic period for AKR mice

period from the time of infection to leukaemia development represents an interval during which changes may be occurring in the lymphocytes of the animal which may be of significance for the final development of neoplasia. This whole period is referred to as the "preleukaemic period" even though on simple morphological grounds the young AKR mouse may not be distinguishable from a normal animal.

In AKR mice an almost unique opportunity is available for studying the progressive changes undergone in a tissue during carcinogenesis. These mice develop leukaemia in 9 out of 10 cases and they can be examined in great detail in the period before leukaemia development with the assurance that some facet of the preleukaemic state is being examined.

Little of significance has been observed in the lymph nodes, spleen and blood of preleukaemic AKR mice. Lymph node and spleen weights are unremarkable and histologically these organs in the preleukaemic period do not appear to differ in structure from those of other mouse strains at the same age. In a comparative study of AKR and C3H mice, higher blood lymphocyte levels were observed in AKR mice than in the low leukaemia strain C3H mice (METCALF and NAKAMURA, 1962). This is reminiscent of the lymphocytosis described in the preleukaemic period in high leukaemia incidence herds of cattle but in mice this relative lymphocytosis is of doubtful significance for other low leukaemia strains of mice, e.g. the C57Bl, have higher blood lymphocyte levels than AKR mice.

The thymus is currently the only organ in preleukaemic AKR mice which has been found to exhibit characteristic preleukaemic changes.

At all ages after birth the AKR thymus is heavier than the thymus in other low leukaemia strains e.g. the C3H. This difference is more obvious in female mice, in which it is also evident that age involution is delayed and less obvious than in male mice or in female mice of other strains. In this regard it is of interest that lymphoid leukaemia occurs earlier and is more frequent in female than in male AKR mice.

In all newborn mice, the thymus cortex exhibits a distinct outer zone, rich in primitive lymphoid cells, which is lost in the first few weeks of life. In AKR mice there is a tendency for the persistence of a distinct, but narrower, peripheral zone of primitive cells throughout adult life.

As was discussed earlier, young adult AKR thymic lymphoid cells proliferate more rapidly than those in other strains and the AKR thymic epithelial and reticulum cells exert a more powerful proliferative stimulus than in other strains (NAKAMURA and METCALF, 1961; METCALF et al., 1961; METCALF, 1962).

Two characteristic morphological changes have been observed in the preleukaemic AKR thymus. These have been briefly described by ARNESEN (1958 a) and SIEGLER and RICH (1963) and examples of these changes are shown in Figs. 38 and 39. The first change we term "*medullary enlargement with cortical thinning*". The overall weight of the thymus showing this change may be normal or slightly subnormal, but there is an absolute increase in the size of the medullary areas which become rounded in outline (NAKAKUKI and NISHIZUKA, 1963). There is an increased number of lymphocytes in the medulla, giving often the appearance of lymphoid follicles. In approximately one third of single sections through AKR thymus glands showing this morphology there are partially developed germinal centres in the medullary collections of lymphoid cells. Such germinal centres contain aggregates of large pyroninophilic cells exhibiting mitotic activity, and between these cells are sometimes phagocytic cells containing lymphocyte debris (METCALF, unpublished data). Plasma cells are fairly numerous in these medullary follicles. The cortex tends to be thinner than

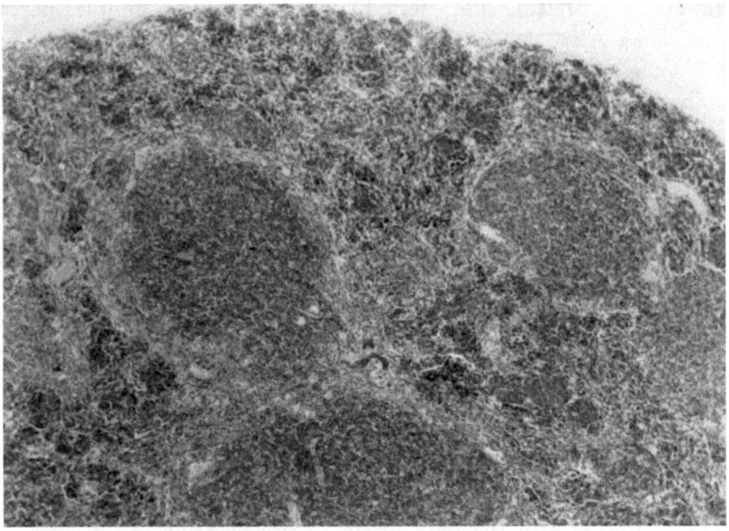

Fig. 38. Section of six months old AKR thymus showing medullary hyperplasia. Note the reduced width of the cortex and the patchy loss of cortical lymphocytes. Medullary areas rounded and enlarged by accumulation of lymphoid cells in follicles. H and E ×80

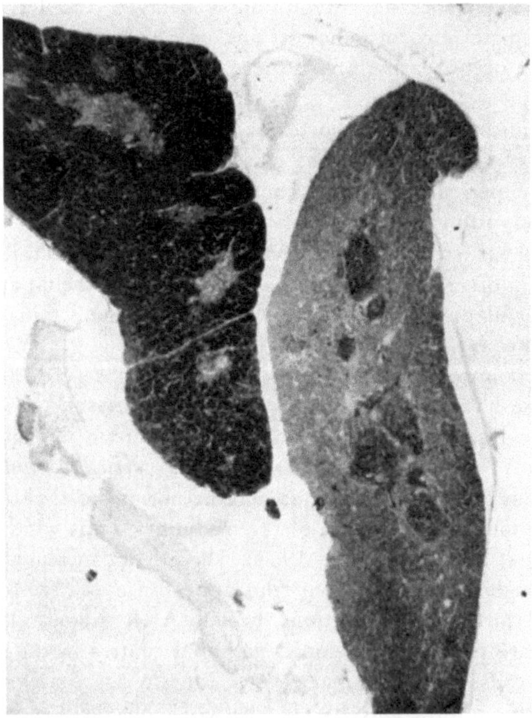

Fig. 39. Low power view of a seven months old AKR thymus with one normal lobe and one lobe showing cortical inversion. Note the loss of cortical lymphoid cells and the medullary areas delineated by lymphocytes surviving from previous medullary lymphoid follicles. H and E ×30

normal and characteristically there is a paucity of small lymphocytes, often focal in nature, giving the cortex an almost "motheaten" appearance. Often the epithelial spaces around the thymic cortical vessels are distended by aggregates of small lymphocytes.

In the second type of preleukaemic change the organ is extremely atrophic and slightly yellowish in colour. Small lymphocytes are virtually absent from the cortex causing a great reduction in cortex volume and a loss of the characteristic dark staining reaction of the cortex in haematoxylin and eosin sections. The medulla is not clearly distinct from the cortex but small areas, which possibly represent the previous sites of lymphoid follicles, are discernable in the medulla because a few small lymphocytes remain in these locations (Fig. 39). This type of thymus has been termed "*cortical inversion*" by us, signifying inversion of the normal appearance in haematoxylin-stained sections due to the greater number of lymphocytes surviving in the medulla than in the cortex. ARNESEN (1958 a) described the medullary epithelial cells as being hyperplastic in preleukamic AKR thymus tissue. It is not clear from the description whether this referred to the medullary enlargement due to lymphoid follicles or to the subsequent uniform appearance of the thymus in cortical inversion, where epithelial cells are very difficult to distinguish from lymphocytes. We have not been convinced that true hypertrophy of the epithelial elements occurs but have noted increased mitotic activity in these cells in the preleukaemic AKR thymus.

The percentage of AKR thymus glands showing these preleukaemic changes at various ages has been determined by killing groups of AKR mice at various ages and is shown in Fig. 40. It will be seen that by six months of age (by which time very few

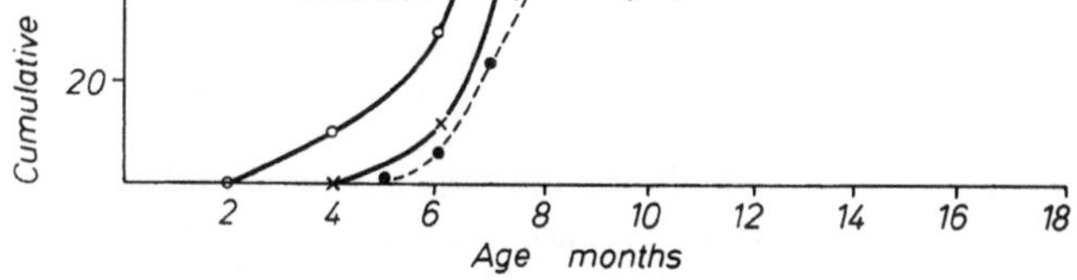

Fig. 40. The incidence at various ages in AKR mice of preleukaemic changes in the thymus. x—x indicates the occurence of microscpic deposits of lymphoma tissue in macroscopically normal thymus glands. Data from 224 AKR mice

AKR mice have developed lymphoid leukaemia) virtually all AKR thymus glands show either medullary enlargement or cortical inversion. It has been pointed out by SIEGLER and RICH (1963), and confirmed by us, that the two thymic lobes (or more properly the two thymus glands) are commonly out of step in developing these preleukaemic changes—one lobe showing medullary enlargement, the other being normal or showing cortical inversion. This fact suggests that neither type of change is likely to be due to a generalised hormonal or environmental influence in the body—but rather to local events occurring asynchronously within the thymic lobes. This is a matter of some importance as the morphological appearance of an AKR thymus with cortical inversion is quite similar to that of the normal thymus after stress or cortisone administration.

Areas of cortical inversion begin in localised areas within the thymus and these spread or coalesce to involve the whole lobe. Areas of cortical inversion are never seen in an otherwise normal thymus, the remainder of the thymus invariably shows medullary enlargement. This suggests that cortical inversion develops secondarily to medullary enlargement.

In this survey of preleukaemic AKR thymus glands, some macroscopically normal thymus glands were found to contain lymphoma tissue. In early cases this lymphoma tissue was in a single focus which was always in the cortex. The remainder of the thymus invariably showed either medullary enlargement or cortical inversion, lymphomata were never seen in an otherwise normal thymus. These relationships are shown diagrammatically in Fig. 41.

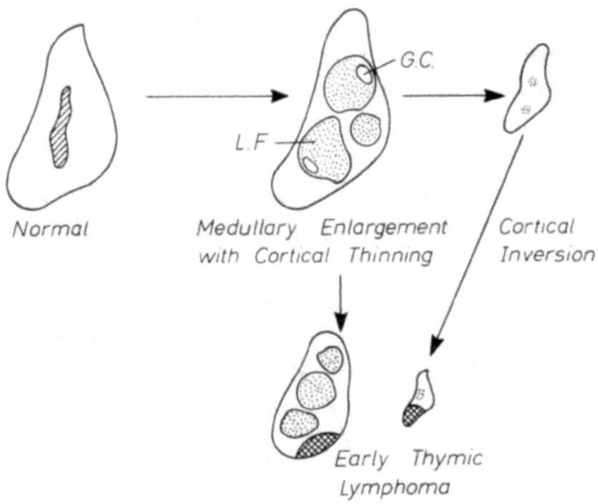

Fig. 41. Schematic diagram of the sequence of thymic morphological changes during leukaemogenesis. Medullary enlargement and cortical thinning precede the development of cortical inversion but lymphomata can develop in thymus glands showing either type of preleukaemic change

The preleukaemic histology of the thymus has not been studied in detail in virus- and chemical carcinogen-induced lymphoid leukaemia. However the author has examined thymus glands kindly made available by Dr. Law, from mice infected with the Moloney lymphoid leukaemia virus and from carcinogen-treated mice. In both, evidence was seen of the occurrence of medullary enlargement and cortical inversion in the preleukaemic period and the situation may be similar in many respects to that described for AKR mice. With Moloney virus, evidence of lymphocyte destruction was frequently very marked, and in the preleukaemic period the cortex frequently contained many phagocytic cells containing pyknotic lymphocytes.

It was shown by Furth and Kahn (1937) that single cells from transplanted leukaemias in AKR mice could be transplanted to normal AKR recipients and there proliferate progressively to kill the recipient animal with transplanted leukaemia. This transplantation procedure can be used as a bioassay to detect the presence of fully developed leukaemic (lymphoma) cells in a tissue under study. In practice, the tissue is minced and injected into young adult recipients which are then observed for some months for the development of transplanted leukaemia. It is doubtful whether the average bioassay test is sensitive enough to detect single lymphoma cells in *spontaneously developing* tumours, as could be demonstrated for passaged lymphoma cells. It seems more likely that the practical limits of detection are probably of the order of 1,000 or more lymphoma cells when using normal recipients and cells from primary lymphomata.

Bioassay tests have been made for the presence of lymphoma cells in AKR thymus glands from preleukaemic mice of various ages, and part of each thymus was examined histologically (METCALF, unpublished data). The thymus tissue was minced and injected intramuscularly into young AKR recipients which were observed for three months for the development of transplanted leukaemia. No transplantable lymphoma cells were demonstrable in thymus glands showing only medullary enlargement or cortical inversion. Those thymus glands showing foci of lymphoma cells gave rise to transplanted tumours (Table 9). The sensitivities of the bioassay procedure and

Table 9. *Comparison of Histological Pattern of Preleukaemic AKR Thymus Glands with Results of Transplantation*

Histological diagnosis	No. of thymus glands tested	No. of thymus glands containing transplantable lymphoma cells
Medullary enlargement	21	0
Cortical inversion	8	0
Early lymphoma	8	7

the histological screening method appeared approximately equal in detecting fully developed lymphoma cells.

The results of this study suggest that fully developed lymphoma cells do not emerge early in the preleukaemic period but only emerge late in the preleukaemic period, after which time the lymphoma cells proliferate at a predictable rate killing the host animal within about four weeks. No evidence was found for the existence of dormant, fully developed, neoplastic cells during the major part of the long (6—8 months) latent period to leukaemia development.

In agreement with the earlier studies of FURTH and BOON (1945), no AKR mice were found in which lymphoma cells were absent from the thymus but were present in other organs—indicating that in most AKR mice the first fully developed lymphoma cells arise in the thymus.

These studies suggest strongly that the development of a lymphoma in the thymus is preceded by a preleukaemic change involving loss of cortical lymphocytes and, initially at least, of medullary enlargement and lymphoid follicle development in the medulla.

The exact nature of the cellular changes in the thymic lymphocyte population during these preleukaemic changes is uncertain. Studies on the mitotic indices of the primitive cells in AKR thymus glands showing medullary hyperplasia indicated that the large and medium lymphoid cells are dividing as rapidly, or possibly even more rapidly, than in either younger AKR thymus glands or the thymus of low leukaemia strain mice of the same age (NAKAMURA and METCALF, 1961). In view of this, the term "preleukaemic atrophy" used by ARNESEN and SIEGLER to describe such thymus glands seems most inappropriate. It was found also that the percentage of primitive lymphoid cells in such thymus glands is higher than normal. The progressive decrease in the percentage of small lymphocytes in the preleukaemic thymus implies either that small lymphocyte production from the mitotic activity of the primitive lymphoid cells is subnormal or that there is an abnormally rapid destruction rate of small lymphocytes. It is tempting to assume that a partial maturation arrest is occurring in the preleukaemic thymus to account for the relative excess of primitive lymphoid cells, as this would form a satisfying intermediate situation between the normal and the neoplastic states. However in view of the weight decrease in the preleukaemic thymus it is probably more likely that the relative deficit of small lymphocytes is due to an excessive destruction rate of these cells, a process which is seen clearly in the Moloney virus infected preleukaemic thymus. Why this excessive destruction of small lymphocytes should be a characteristic event in the preleukaemic period is difficult to see but its occurrence is invariable and it must therefore bear some relationship to leukaemogenesis.

It was previously noted that PAS-positive reticulum cells of the thymus cortex are related in some way with the mitotic activity of adjacent thymic lymphocytes. This phenomenon is more marked in the preleukaemic AKR thymus than in other strains and more marked in AKR thymus glands showing medullary enlargement or cortical inversion than in the young AKR thymus (METCALF and ISHIDATE, 1962). The significance of this observation is not clear. It could indicate the existence of some type of virus-induced disturbance of the relationship between PAS cells and lymphocytes as postulated earlier, or it may merely be the result of lymphocyte destruction in the AKR thymus with an abortive attempt at thymus regeneration, for the PAS cell—mitotic lymphocyte association is more marked in the regenerating thymus (ISHIDATE and METCALF, 1963).

3. Analysis of Sequential Preleukaemic Changes

The morphological changes in the preleukaemic thymus are capable of further analysis by the use of thymus grafts. As has been discussed, it is difficult to obtain satisfactory grafts using old donor animals. Despite this limitation, we have examined the morphology of 7 months old AKR thymus glands, showing either medullary enlargement or cortical inversion, one month after grafting to two months old young adult AKR mice. This study revealed that the preleukaemic thymus grafts showed the same morphological abnormalities (medullary enlargement with lymphoid follicles and lymphocyte stasis, or cortical inversion) as did the donor thymus (METCALF, unpublished data). However when day old AKR thymus glands were grafted to seven or eight months old AKR recipients, these grafts a month later had attained normal size and showed quite normal morphology despite the fact that the host thymus showed preleukaemic changes, and in one or two cases actually had early lymphomata (Fig. 42). Bearing in mind the fact that donor epithelial and reticulum cells survive in thymus grafts, but that the lymphoid cells are replaced by host cells, these results imply that the epithelial and reticulum cell elements of the thymus may be responsible for the observed morphological preleukaemic changes in the cortical lymphoid population, and that if the epithelial and reticulum cells are abnormal, the normal young adult cells which repopulate the grafts may be made to behave abnormally.

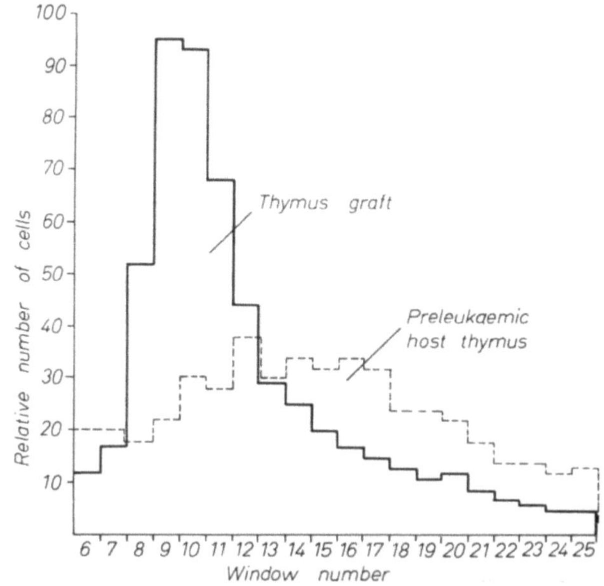

Fig. 42. Coulter counter analysis of cell populations in host thymus and thymus graft in an 8 months old AKR mouse grafted one month previously with a day old AKR thymus gland. Host thymus exhibited cortical inversion and tracing shows an absence of the small lymphocyte peak present in normal thymus tissue and an increased content of medium and large cells. In contrast, the thymus graft exhibited normal morphology in section and the cell distribution pattern is that of normal thymus tissue

These graft findings, implicating the epithelial and reticulum cells as the cell system in which progressive preleukaemic changes occur, are at variance with other experimental data which suggest that the lymphocyte population is the one developing preleukaemic changes. When AKR spleen cell suspensions of various ages were injected into baby (AKR × C3H)F_1 mice, it was found that these mice subsequently developed thymic and generalised leukaemia and many of these leukaemias were demonstrated by transplantation tests to have originated from the injected AKR cells (Metcalf, 1962; Metcalf, 1963 a). Somewhat similar results were reported by Lorenz, Law and Congdon (1954) who showed that AKR bone marrow cells injected into (C3H × AKR)F_1 mice seeded in the host organs and later became neoplastic. Several points of importance were demonstrated in these experiments. First, spleen and bone marrow cells were capable of seeding in the thymus and there becoming neoplastic, probably confirming the normal occurrence of cell migration streams from the bone marrow and spleen to the thymus. Second, it was apparent in these experiments that preleukaemic changes had occurred in the spleen cells before they were injected into the recipient mice. The older the cells used, the shorter was the latent period to leukaemia development in the new host. In fact the latent interval to development of neoplasia in the injected spleen cells was that which would have occurred if these cells had been left in the donor animals. This strongly suggests that age-related preleukaemic changes do develop in the lymphoid cells (or whichever spleen cells repopulate the thymus).

These experiments also raise the possibility that despite the fact that the first fully developed leukaemic cells appear in the thymus, the *initial* preleukaemic changes in the lymphoid cells may occur in some site other than the thymus—specifically in the spleen or bone marrow. If this is so it may explain one of the puzzling features of the distribution of leukaemia viruses—at least in preleukaemic AKR mice—namely, that viral particles are more readily observable in spleen and bone marrow cells than in thymic cells.

Further evidence for the development of sequential preleukaemic changes in lymphoid populations was obtained when it was shown that six month old AKR spleen cells are no longer in a thymus-dependent state, but in a thymus-responsive state (METCALF, 1962 a). Since thymectomy at the age of two months prevents lymphoid leukaemia development, the thymus is necessary if the lymphoid cells of two months old AKR mice are to progress to neoplasia. In the terminology of endocrine organ carcinogenesis, this would represent a "thymus dependent" phase in the sequence from normal lymphocyte to leukaemic cell. It was found that six month old preleukaemic spleen cells would develop into leukaemic cells when injected into thymectomised (AKR $\times$ C3H)F_1 recipients—that is, in the absence of a thymic influence. However the latent period to leukaemia development for these injected cells was longer than when spleen cells from the same donors were injected into sham operated (AKR $\times$ C3H)F_1 recipients. This would correspond to a "thymus responsive" phase in the leukaemogenesis sequence. As discussed earlier, fully developed leukaemic cells are "autonomous" with respect to the thymus and grow equally rapidly in thymectomised and normal mice. These data indicate that lymphoid leukaemogenesis shares features in common with the classically established sequence for endocrine tumourigenesis, where the target cells becoming neoplastic pass through three states—dependency, responsiveness and autonomy—with respect to the specific stimulating endocrine influence. In the context of lymphoid leukaemogenesis, the lymphoid population appears to pass through stages of dependency on the thymus, to responsiveness to the thymus to autonomy to the thymus.

It is of some interest that cytological and autoradiographic analyses have shown that thymic lymphoma cells divide more slowly than normal thymic lymphoid cells in AKR mice (NAKAMURA and METCALF, 1961; METCALF and WIADROWSKI, 1966). It has also been found that, unlike the situtation with normal thymic and lymph node lymphocyte division rates, the rate of division of thymic lymphoma cells is no higher than that of the lymph node lymphoma cells in the same animal (METCALF, NAKAMURA and WIADROWSKI, 1965). These results imply that when lymphoma cells become autonomous with respect to the thymic influence, they also lose their responsiveness to stimulation by the intrinsic thymic proliferative stimulus.

No investigations appear to have been carried out to determine whether or not lymphoma cells are responsive to stimulation by foreign antigens, as are normal lymphoid cells, but such information would be of considerable interest.

There is some evidence therefore that sequential changes occur in the preleukaemic period and that these changes may occur in both the lymphoid population (the cell population becoming neoplastic) and in the thymic epithelial and reticulum cells (the cell population possibly influencing the development of neoplastic changes in the lymphoid cells).

4. Thymic Humoral Influence in Leukaemogenesis

Since it is now established that part at least of the thymic influence on lymphopoiesis and immune responses is mediated via a humoral factor, it is legitimate to raise the question of whether or not the thymic influence on lymphoid leukaemia development is mediated by a humoral factor.

As has been shown, lymphoid leukaemic cells characteristically first appear inside the thymus itself. When thymus grafts restore susceptibility to lymphoid leukaemia development, it is again usual to find that the thymus is the site of initiation of the leukaemic process. This suggests the operation of a short range influence (either cell contact or special microenvironment) as the inductive influence exerted by the thymus on lymphoid cells in leukaemia development, rather than the operation of a simple thymic humoral factor. However it can be argued that the thymus may induce neoplastic change in lymphoid cells via a humoral factor, and since this factor probably would be at its highest concentration in the thymus, this fact alone would account for the almost invariable location of the original neoplastic change in the thymus itself.

A somewhat different effect of thymus grafting from the usual results (primary graft lymphomata) was observed in studies on the effect of thymus grafting to leukaemia resistant F_1 hybrids resulting from crosses between high and low leukaemia strains of mice. When AKR thymus grafts were placed subcutaneously in (AKR $\times$ C57Bl)F_1 mice, the incidence of lymphoid leukaemia was raised from 9% to 20%. In addition, the incidence of reticulum cell sarcoma was increased from 27% to 47% (METCALF, 1964 b). In only two cases did the thymus graft appear to be the site of origin of neoplasia development in these animals and in one of these two cases it was demonstrated that the neoplastic cells were F_1 host in origin. When the generalised lymphoid leukaemias and reticulum cell sarcomata arising in the thymus-grafted animals were tested, all were found to have originated from F_1 host cells.

Similar results were reported by NAKAKUKI and NISHIZUKA (1962) who grafted AKR thymus glands subcutaneously to leukaemia resistant (A/Jax $\times$ AKR)F_1 mice. Again the incidence of generalised lymphoid leukaemia and reticulum cell sarcoma was elevated but only one leukaemic tumour arose in the graft site.

It is evident from these data in leukaemia resistant F_1 mice that AKR thymus grafts can sometimes induce neoplastic transformation in host cells under conditions in which the cells apparently do not need to be within the graft itself to undergo neoplastic transformation. These experiments suggest that a humoral factor may be involved in leukaemogenesis and raise the interesting possibility that a thymic humoral influence may be involved also in reticulum cell sarcoma development.

It should be possible to prove or disprove the existence of a leukaemogenic thymic humoral factor by the use of thymus graft tissue in millipore diffusion chambers—the technique so successfully used to prove the existence of the thymic humoral factor influencing immune responses. So far as the author is aware no successful experiment has been carried out using thymus tissue in diffusion chambers to restore susceptibility to lymphoid leukaemia, although this experiment has been attempted in thymectomised, virus-injected and thymectomised, irradiated mice and lately by ourselves in thymectomised, high leukaemia strain (AKR × C3H)F_1 mice (METCALF, WIADROWSKI and BRADLEY, 1965). However it cannot be concluded from the failures so far that a thymic factor is not involved in leukaemogenesis. One serious technical problem exists in the leukaemogenesis studies which was not of importance in the studies on the restoration of immune competence. In the diffusion chambers presently in use, thymus tissue survival is relatively poor and it is highly doubtful whether adequate amounts of viable tissue (even epithelial and reticulum cells) survive for more than a few weeks. The restoration of immune competence by thymic humoral factor merely requires the presence of humoral factor for a few days, and this is readily achieved with existing chambers. If leukaemogenesis requires the constant production of humoral factor for several months, this cannot be achieved with present diffusion chambers, so it still is not possible to be dogmatic on whether a thymic humoral factor is, or is not, relevant for leukaemogenesis. We, and others, also have failed to confer susceptibility to lymphoid leukaemia development by giving repeated injections of thymus extract but again these experiments cannot positively exclude the operation of a humoral factor for little of this factor may be stored within the thymus itself, and thymus extracts may be poor in humoral factor or even contain an inhibitor of humoral factor.

During the work in our laboratory on the lymphocytosis stimulating effects of thymus extracts in baby mice, a considerable amount of work was done on the activity of material from preleukaemic and leukaemic mice. It was found that serum from normal mice did not elicit a lymphocytosis in injected mice, but serum from preleukaemic AKR and C58 mice aged 2—6 months did do so, as also did serum from AKR mice with lymphoid leukaemia. Thymectomy of preleukaemic AKR mice removed detectable serum activity when the animals were tested three months later. Thymus extracts from preleukaemic and neoplastic AKR thymus tissue induced a lymphocytosis and there was some evidence that seven day old AKR thymus glands contained more lymphocytosis stimulating factor than did the C3H or C57Bl thymus from mice of the same age (METCALF, 1959 a).

As with the results from tests on normal mouse organ extracts, it was found that, in leukaemic mice, only thymic lymphoma extracts exhibited activity, and extracts made of lymphoma deposits in other organs were without activity (METCALF, 1956 b). When thymic lymphoma tissue was transplanted to normal recipients, and allowed to proliferate until the recipient animals were moribund, the transplanted lymphoma tissue exhibited no lymphocytosis stimulating activity.

These results suggest that the thymic epithelial and reticulum cells of preleukaemic mice may secrete excessive amounts of LSF which enters the serum in such quantities as to be detectable by the rather crude bioassay system used. The LSF activity demonstrated in primary thymic lymphoma tissue may be due to the survival of epithelial and reticulum cells scattered amongst the mass of lymphoma cells. Since the epithelial and reticulum cells are in general non-dividing cells, they may have been diluted out during the growth of the transplanted thymic lymphoma tissue, leading to a loss of detectable LSF in this tissue.

It is not certain whether the intrinsic thymic proliferative stimulus is identical with LSF, but the thymus graft data described earlier indicate that AKR thymic epithelial and reticulum cells exert a stronger proliferative stimulus on repopulating cells than do low leukaemia strain C3H cells.

These observations suggest that the thymus in preleukaemic and leukaemic mice may be functionally overactive and may tend to stimulate excessive lymphopoiesis in the preleukaemic period. This excessive lymphopoiesis is most evident in the thymus itself (NAKAMURA and METCALF, 1961).

As was pointed out by KAPLAN, NAGAREDA and BROWN (1954) factors tending to increase lymphopoiesis also increase the incidence of lymphoid leukaemia in mice, and vice versa. If, as now seems likely, a thymic humoral factor plays an important role in the regulation of lymphopoiesis, it is significant that levels of thymic LSF are elevated in preleukaemic AKR and C58 mice and in mice subjected to whole body irradiation in leukaemogenic doses (METCALF, 1959; 1959 a).

In view of what is now known of the role of leukaemia viruses in leukaemogenesis, and the strong suggestion that local intrathymic factors are of importance in leukaemogenesis, it is doubtful whether the thymic influence in lymphoid leukaemia development is solely mediated through a humoral factor, but such a factor might well play an important accessory role in the development of the disease.

Most of what is known of the pathogenesis of lymphoid leukaemia has been derived from studies in mice and rats, and it is uncertain whether any of the processes demonstrated have any relevance for an understanding of the development of human leukaemia. The classical type lymphoid leukaemia in the mouse does not correspond exactly to the usual forms of either acute or chronic lymphoid leukaemia in humans. Occasional children with acute leukaemia do exhibit a disease pattern identical with the mouse disease, complete to the large thymic lymphoma, but such cases are exceptional. However, it is of some interest that histologically, mouse lymphoma tissue is identical in morphology with that of the Burkitt lymphoma tissue from Africa and New Guinea and with occasional lymphosarcomata occurring in other countries.

It is of some interest therefore that the baby mouse bioassay system has revealed evidence of lymphocytosis stimulating activity in sera from human cases of chronic lymphatic leukaemia and lymphosarcoma. A survey made of serum activity from patients with various types of leukaemia and reticular tumours revealed that lymphocytosis stimulating activity could be demonstrated in virtually all cases of chronic lymphatic leukaemia and lymphosarcoma but no similar activity was demonstrable in sera from cases of acute lymphoid leukaemia. Similarly sera from acute and chronic myeloid leukaemia and Hodgkin's disease were inactive as were sera from a variety of other haematological or neoplastic diseases (METCALF, 1956, 1956 a). So far as could be determined, the lymphocytosis stimulating factor in human leukaemic serum appeared to be similar to, if not identical with, thymic LSF and certainly the injection of human leukaemic sera into baby mice affected thymic LSF activity in these mice in the same way as did injections of thymic LSF (METCALF, 1956 b). In three cases of chronic lymphoid leukaemia in humans, local irradiation over the thymus region appeared to depress serum lymphocytosis stimulating activity (METCALF, unpublished data).

These studies in humans are in urgent need of confirmation but if they prove correct, they imply that a thymic humoral factor may be involved in chronic lymphoid leukaemia and lymphosarcoma, although strangely enough, not in acute lymphoid leukaemia in man.

It is of some interest that chromosome studies on chronic lymphoid leukaemic cells have failed so far to reveal the anticipated chromosome abnormalities typical of neoplastic cells e.g. as in acute leukaemia. The protracted course of chronic lymphoid leukaemia has raised in the past the question of whether this disease may not be a neoplastic one but rather a severe and long lasting disturbance of lymphocyte homeostasis (possibly sometimes terminating in true neoplasia). If this suggestion has any truth, it may well be that the thymus and a thymic humoral factor could be implicated in the development of the disease.

Recently GRUTER, TRAPP and SANGER (1965) have reported that sera from patients with Mongolism produce a lymphocytosis when injected intracerebrally into baby mice. This observation is of interst in view of the predisposition of patients with Mongolism to develop leukaemia.

5. Immune Status of Preleukaemic Mice

Some mention needs to be made of special immune responses occurring in mice during leukaemogenesis, of the possible involvement of the thymus in such processes and of the possible importance these immune responses may have for leukaemogenesis itself.

It has now been shown that AKR lymphoma cells or lymphoma cells induced by the Gross virus in other mouse strains contain a new antigen not present in the normal animal (SLETTENMARK and KLEIN, 1962). This antigen may, or may not, be identical with the antigen of the Gross virus itself. More recently OLD, BOYSE and STOCKERT (1965) have shown the presence of this antigen (the G antigen) in the lymphoid tissues of normal young adult AKR mice, presumably as a consequence of the prenatal infection of these mice by the Gross virus. This G antigen is not strong but animals can be immunised against it and will then reject challenge grafts of isologous lymphoma cells. One might wonder therefore why an AKR mouse does not develop an immune response against the G antigen, and as a consequence, eliminate the first few emerging antigenic lymphoma cells, thereby preventing leukaemia development.

It now appears that the AKR mouse is specifically tolerant of the G antigen and cannot be immunised against it (AXELRAD, 1965). It is likely that the basis for this tolerance is exposure of the AKR mouse to the antigen (in the form of viral antigen or antigen from virally modified host cells) in foetal life—at which time this foreign antigen is still acceptable to the animal as "self" antigen.

The mechanisms underlying the recognition of "self" and "non-self" antigens are not fully understood and it is not known what role the thymus plays in this continuing process. If the thymus is involved in "non-self" recognition, it could be postulated that the AKR thymus may exert a leukaemogenic influence by its failure to generate cells with the capacity to initiate an immune rejection response to cells (including lymphoma cells) carrying the G antigen. Such a postulated function for the thymus is actually quite unlikely in the development of lymphoid leukaemia for on this basis, thymectomy of low leukaemia strain mice should render them susceptible to lymphoid leukaemogenesis, whereas of course thymectomy actually prevents lymphoid leukaemia development in all mouse strains.

Indeed, as was discussed earlier, the thymus has been shown to break down the tolerant state and thus an AKR animal should have a greater chance of becoming "non tolerant" and possibly of eliminating infection by the Gross leukaemia virus or eliminating lymphoma cells containing the G antigen (thus *preventing* leukaemia development) if the thymus is present rather than if thymectomy is performed.

It was reported by PETERSON, HENDRICKSON and GOOD (1963) and DENT, PETERSON and GOOD (1965) that C3H mice injected with passaged GROSS leukaemia virus exhibited depressed immune responses and a depressed capacity to reject Ce/J skin grafts (same H_2 locus). They suggested that a generalised depression of immune responses may be a significant feature of the preleukaemic animal.

However preleukaemic AKR mice appear to react normally to other antigens e.g. sheep red cells, and no evidence has been obtained that preleukaemic AKR mice exhibit abnormal immune reactivity to antigens other than the lymphoma virus/cell G antigen (METCALF, unpublished data).

6. Is Leukaemogenesis due to an Intrathymic Breakdown in Immune Tolerance?

It can be seen from the foregoing discussion that although much has been learned of why the thymus is necessary for lymphoid leukaemia development, something of a stalemate has developed. There is evidence to implicate a leukaemia virus in leukaemogenesis and evidence that, the more virus that is present, the more rapid is leukaemia development. On the host cell side, there is evidence that the more rapidly the lymphoid cells divide, the greater the incidence of leukaemia. The present concept held by most workers of the role of the thymus in the development of lymphoid leukaemia seems to hover uncertainly between postulating that the thymus has a higher (critical) content of virus than other tissues and/or that thymic cells are peculiarly susceptible to neoplastic change because they are special cells, because of their rapid rate of division or because large aggregates of susceptible primitive lymphoid cells exist in juxtaposition to virus in the thymus.

In considering this situation, we have been struck by two puzzling features.

1. Why is there such a long latent period to leukaemia development (in AKR mice) when virus and rapidly dividing primitive lymphoid cells presumably are present in the thymus at birth? Why is it not until middle age that the first leukaemic cells develop?

2. If the thymus is the fulcrum of the body's immune defence system against foreign antigens, why should the thymus be *necessary* for the emergence and proliferation of leukaemic cells which are known to be antigenic and which should be the target of a thymus-directed immune rejection response?

We have been impressed by the fact that tolerance to the leukaemia virus antigen can be demonstrated in mice infected neonatally by leukaemia virus. This emphasises some remarkable similarities which exist between tolerance breakdown and lymphoid leukaemia induction. Thymectomy slows or prevents tolerance breakdown and leukaemia development, whereas thymus grafting and irradiation accelerate tolerance breakdown and increase susceptibility to leukaemia development.

This has prompted us to construct a new hypothesis for the role of the thymus in the development of lymphoid leukaemia which is not necessarily exclusive of any of the foregoing proposals advanced to explain the role of the thymus in this disease, but which takes into account the immune reactivity of the animal during leukaemogenesis.

It is proposed that following prenatal or neonatal infection by the leukaemia virus, a state of tolerance develops to the foreign antigen of the leukaemia virus. Infection of host tissues is widespread and the situation is exactly comparable with the asymptomatic state existing in neonatal lymphocytic choriomeningitis infection in mice. Lymphoid leukaemia arises because of a sequence of events initiated by a breakdown in tolerance to the virus which occurs *locally* within the thymus. A local cellular immune response develops in the thymus and as a result of interaction between the immunologically active cells and the virus infected lymphoid cells, many of the latter are destroyed. However occasional virus infected lymphoid cells are not destroyed but become altered in such a way as to become neoplastic lymphoid cells. These cells are relatively insusceptible to further damage by the immunologically active cells and proliferate freely, ultimately killing the host animal with generalised lymphoid leukaemia. This proposal is shown diagrammatically in Figure 43. Essen-

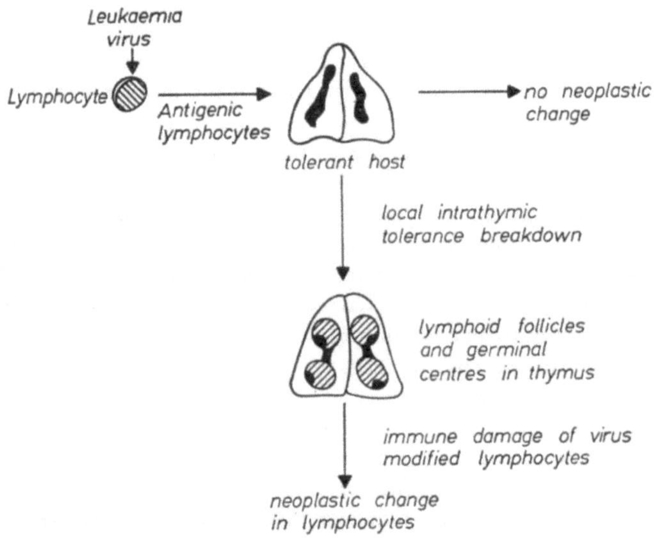

Fig. 43. Schematic diagram of proposed events during leukaemogenesis. Neonatal infection of lymphoid cells by Gross virus leads to a tolerant state and no disease development. Following local breakdown in tolerance in the thymus to the G antigen, foci of immunologically active cells develop in the medulla. The immune rejection response developing in the thymus leads to destruction of cortical lymphocytes carrying the G antigen but surviving damaged lymphoid cells may either be leukaemic cells or be specially prone subsequently to become neoplastic

tially this proposal suggests that the leukaemia virus does not induce leukaemia by a direct action on host cells, but rather that leukaemia results when a host immune response produces secondary damage in virus infected cells.

How does this proposal fit the facts established about lymphoid leukaemia development? As has been recounted, the leukaemia virus and leukaemia virus infected cells have been shown to contain an antigen foreign to the host animal. However AKR mice, infected with this virus in the prenatal period, are tolerant to this antigen and cannot be immunised against it in early life. The thymus is known to break down tolerance to foreign antigens and thymectomy is known to delay or prevent tolerance breakdown. Tolerance may be broken down more rapidly in thymectomised animals by thymus grafting. On the basis of the present hypothesis, thymectomy, by delaying breakdown in tolerance to the leukaemia virus, would prevent or reduce lymphoid leukaemia development whilst thymus grafting would restore the animal's ability to break down the tolerant state and so restore susceptibility to lymphoid leukaemia development.

Why is it postulated that the breakdown in the tolerant state is *local* and restricted to within the thymus itself? The characteristic feature of the preleukaemic AKR thymus is the development of lymphoid follicles and sometimes germinal centres in the thymic medulla itself. No other obvious changes have been observed in other AKR tissues at this time. Such lymphoid follicles are the classical morphological expression of a local immune response. Associated with this appearance of medullary lymphoid follicles is a progressive depletion of lymphoid cells from the thymus cortex. An autoradiographic analysis of the lymphoid cell kinetics in such thymus glands has suggested that the primitive cells are proliferating at a normal rate but that there is an excessively rapid destruction of small lymphocytes (METCALF and WIADROWSKI, unpublished data). This would be compatible with a situation where lymphocytes were being destroyed by an immune rejection process. However when neonatal thymus grafts are placed in preleukaemic AKR mice, the grafts, although repopulated by host lymphoid cells have a normal morphology with normal thymic lymphopoiesis and differentiation, and a normal rate of destruction of small lymphocytes. This fact is against the presence of circulating antibodies in the preleukaemic animal and implies that if an immune response is occurring against virus-infected lymphoid cells, it is restricted to the host thymus and is a local, cell-mediated, immune response.

In the earlier discussion on the role played by the thymus in breaking tolerance it was concluded that the thymus either generates new cells capable of reacting with the antigen concerned or more likely, provides a humoral factor activating newly created lymphoid cells, possibly originating from the bone marrow, to initiate an active immune response. On either basis, given the existence of the antigen within the thymus itself, it would be reasonable to expect that an immune response would occur first in the thymus medulla, either because the cells were generated in the thymus or because extrathymic cells entering the medulla would be exposed to a higher concentration of humoral factor in the thymic medulla than anywhere else in the body. The local nature of the breakdown in tolerance would explain one characteristic feature of leukaemogenesis, that the first accumulation of lymphoma cells arises in the thymus itself or in the thymus graft in thymectomised animals.

The AKR thymus produces more humoral factor (LSF) than does the thymus in other strains. If this humoral factor represents the humoral factor breaking tolerance, then AKR thymus grafts in thymectomised (AKR $\times$ C3H)F_1 hybrids would be more likely to induce leukaemia than C3H thymus grafts since they produce higher levels of humoral factor.

In this hypothesis a mouse strain like the C57Bl is conceived of as also being infected by leukaemia virus but as being in a permanently tolerant state. Whole body irradiation might then be expected to produce leukaemia because of its known ability to accelerate or precipitate tolerance breakdown, possibly by stimulating an increased thymic production of humoral factor (cf. the evidence of METCALF [1959] and ITO and WEINSTEIN [1962] on elevated serum LSF levels in irradiated animals). On the same basis, thymectomy coupled with irradiation might prevent leukaemia development by again preventing tolerance breakdown. Possibly, grafting a C57Bl thymus graft to a thymectomised (AKR × C57Bl)F_1 mouse might not restore susceptibility to lymphoid leukaemia development because the grafting of a thymus from a tolerant animal to a thymectomised recipient might allow tolerance to persist (cf. the experiments of ISAKOVIC, SMITH and WAKSMAN, 1965).

The role of the dose level of virus in an animal in shortening the latent period (accelerating tolerance breakdown) is uncertain, particularly since the more antigen that is present in an animal the more likely it should be that tolerance will *persist*. However it may be that virus-infected host cells are more susceptible to immune reaction damage if the level of virus-infectivity is high. The high level of virus (antigen) in the thymus might also tend to make an immune response more likely to be initiated in the thymus than elsewhere.

The observation that factors increasing lymphopoiesis tend to increase the incidence of lymphoid leukaemia might be explained on the basis that the higher the rate of lymphopoiesis in the animal, the more likely that cells with new reactivity patterns will be generated in the tolerant animal, which will then be capable of mounting an immune response against the viral antigen.

This hypothesis could be developed at greater length to account for some of the other observations on leukaemogenesis in mice but the important feature of the proposal is that it lends itself to experimental verification. If this concept is correct it should be possible, in preleukaemic AKR mice in which the thymus exhibits medullary lymphoid follicles, to demonstrate the presence of cells in the thymus which are capable of reacting against either leukaemia virus or leukaemia virus-infected cells (e.g. young adult AKR lymph node cells) using established techniques for demonstrating *in vitro* cytotoxic effects. Such cells should not be present in the very young AKR thymus for this animal is in a tolerant state. Such cells may also be absent from the tissues of mice with established lymphoid leukaemia for it has been shown that leukaemic mice are capable of mounting only weak immune responses to foreign antigens (METCALF, unpublished data) either because the normal lymphoid tissues have been replaced by lymphoma cells or because lymphoma cell invasion has disrupted the vital network of antigen trapping and processing reticuloendothelial cells. For the reasons advanced earlier it seems unlikely that circulating antibodies would be present in preleukaemic mice.

This postulated breakdown in the preleukaemic period of tolerance to the leukaemia virus antigen, although normally restricted to the thymus might also occur more slowly in other tissues for example, the spleen. This might account for the late development of lymphoid leukaemia and reticulum cell sarcoma in some thymectomised animals. Certainly we have been struck by the pronounced reticulo-endothelial cell hyperplasia in the spleens of old thymectomised AKR and AKR F_1 hybrid mice and this might represent a slowly progressive cellular immune response against leukaemia virus antigen of the same type as been postulated to develop earlier, and more readily, in the thymus.

The concept that neoplastic cells arise when cells escape from a potentially lethal environment is not new. This concept has frequently been advanced in chemical carcinogenesis (e.g. carcinogenesis with cytotoxic drugs) where the chemicals concerned are exhibiting low grade toxic effects on the tissues and where the possibility exists that cells able to modify their metabolism in such a way as to escape these toxic effects are either neoplastic cells or are likely to become neoplastic cells.

Possibly this present proposal for the role of the thymus in lymphoid leukaemia development will be shown to be erroneous by future investigations. However it has one virtue in explaining the paradoxical situation which has arisen from the demonstration that the thymus regulates and directs immune responses against foreign antigens, but that the thymus is necessary for the emergence and proliferation of leukaemic cells which are known to contain foreign antigens—the very situation in which a thymus directed immune response should be most effective in preventing disease development.

Summary

Thymectomy prevents lymphoid leukaemia development in mice and thymus grafts restore susceptibility to leukaemia development, whether this be of the spontaneous type, or induced by virus, chemicals or irradiation. The thymus from some strains of mice can confer susceptibility to lymphoid leukaemia whilst the thymus from others cannot.

The development of lymphoid leukaemia in a lymphoid cell population is a stepwise process in which the lymphoid cells pass through phases of dependency, responsiveness and autonomy with respect to the thymic influence. The initial phases of this sequence may occur in cells located elsewhere in the body which later seed in the thymus and there finally acquire the full characteristics of neoplastic cells.

The thymic influence appears to be positive rather than negative and to be exerted by the epithelial and reticulum cell elements of the thymus. However the intrinsic susceptibility of the thymic lymphoid cells to neoplastic change appears to influence the length of the latent period to leukaemia development and possibly the final incidence of lymphoid leukaemia.

The nature of the thymic influence is uncertain. There is some evidence for the presence of excess levels of thymic humoral factor in preleukaemic and leukaemic mice but attempts to induce lymphoid leukaemia with thymus grafts in diffusion chambers or with thymus extracts so far have been unsuccessful. The thymus may harbour usually high levels of leukaemia virus, a situation which may be essential if neoplasia is to occur in lymphoid cells infected by these virus particles, or alternatively the lymphoid leukaemia viruses may operate indirectly by infecting the non-lymphoid thymic cells, leading to subsequent changes in the regulation by these cells of lymphocyte proliferation and differentiation. Thymic lymphoid cells may be particularly susceptible to neoplastic change possibly because they proliferate more rapidly than other lymphoid cells or possibly because they are a unique type of lymphoid cell.

It is possible that lymphoid leukaemia develops because of a local intrathymic breakdown of tolerance to the leukaemia virus antigen and that leukaemia is not the direct result of virus infection of lymphoid cells but the result of secondary immune damage to virus infected cells.

Chapter 9

The Thymus and Carcinogenesis

Passing from the special relationship between the thymus and lymphoid leukaemia development, we must now discuss the question of whether or not the thymus has any influence on the development and growth of other types of cancer.

From the preceding discussion of the function of the thymus, it is obvious that the thymus could influence tumour development:

1. by affecting host immune responses particularly when the emerging tumour cells are antigenic for the host, and/or 2. by producing some factor having a trophic effect for tumour cells or having a modifying effect on the nutritional or metabolic state of the animal which favours tumour cell growth.

Before discussing what is known of the effect of the thymus on carcinogenesis it is necessary to consider whether any, or all, tumour cells contain new antigens not present in the host animal and whether such antigenic cells might provoke significant immune responses in the host.

The subject of tumour antigens is rather confused but has been summarised admirably in two recent reviews by DAY (1965) and HELLSTROM and MOLLER (1965). Examples have now been documented of tumours which have acquired new antigens, lost normal antigens, have normal antigens in excessive amounts, have normal antigens belonging to organs other than the organ of origin of the tumour or have antigens present in the tumour which are present in the tissue of origin in the embryonic state, but not in adult life. Of these various situations the one of special interest to a discussion of the role of the thymus in carcinogenesis is the situation in which tumour cells contain a new antigen not present in the normal animal.

The first example of this occurrence was described by FOLEY (1953) and confirmed by PREHN and MAIN (1957). These workers showed that methyl-cholanthrene induced sarcomata in C3H mice could be resected and after irradiation used to immunise either the original host animal or other mice of the same strain. These immunised animals were then found to be capable of rejecting challenge transplants of the sarcoma used for immunisation. This tumour immunity was specific for individual sarcomata (PREHN and MAIN, 1957; KLEIN et al., 1960; OLD et al., 1962), and an animal immunised against one sarcoma was not resistant to challenge transplants of other methylcholanthrene induced sarcomata arising in mice of the same strain. The basis for this phenomenon appears to be the development of a new antigen in the sarcoma cells which is recognisable by the host as being foreign and which is capable, when presented in a suitable form, of eliciting a homograft immune response which allows the animal to reject challenge transplants of a limited number of sarcoma cells bearing the same antigen. It is important to emphasize that this type of host immunity is not all-powerful, for if sufficient tumour cells are transplanted, the immune defences can be broken down and the animal succumbs from a progressively growing tumour. This comment applies to all the examples of tumour immunity to be described. A delicate balance usually exists between emerging antigenic tumour cells and the antigen-stimulated host defences, a balance which can easily be upset in favour of the emerging tumour cells. Provided only a few tumour cells are present they can be suppressed or killed by the host, but should tumour cell proliferation be rapid, breakthrough of the host's immune defence system is possible. Obviously the more strongly antigenic a tumour cell is, the more chance the host has of mounting an effective immune response, and the weaker the antigens the less effective will be the resulting immune response. Thus GLOBERSON and FELDMAN (1964 a) observed that the capacity for growth of primary transplants from sarcomata produced in C3H and C57Bl mice by benzopyrene was determined by the intrinsic antigenicity of the tumour cells themselves.

Subsequent to this work on chemically-induced tumours, it was shown that viral-induced tumours also contain foreign antigens which elicit host immune responses capable of eliminating or suppressing tumour cells containing these antigens. The basic system used is to infect an animal with a tumour virus and show that this animal will later reject challenge transplants from tumours induced by the same virus. In this case the viral-induced tumours differ from the carcinogen-induced tumours in containing group-specific antigens, not tumour-specific antigens. For example, in all lymphomata induced by the Gross virus it can be shown that the cells contain a similar antigen which when used to immunise animals will protect them against challenge transplants of all lymphomata induced by this virus.

The tumour viruses which induce foreign antigen development in tumour cells include the polyoma virus (SJOGREN, HELLSTROM and KLEIN, 1961; HABEL, 1962), SV40 (HABEL and EDDY, 1963; KOCH and SABIN, 1963; DEFENDI, 1963) and the leukaemia viruses (SLETTENMARK and KLEIN, 1962; KLEIN, SJOGREN and KLEIN, 1962). Basically it is possible to have two types of foreign antigen in such tumour cells 1. tumour virus antigen either in the form of infectious virus or masked viral antigen perhaps combined with the host cell genome, or 2. foreign antigen, not related to viral antigen, but produced by the infected host cell as a specific response to infection by the tumour virus.

With polyoma virus there is now good evidence for the existence of both types of antigen, but in the case of the lymphomata induced by the Gross and Moloney leukaemia viruses, it is still uncertain whether only viral antigen is involved or whether there is also a host cell-produced foreign antigen. Certainly animals may be immunised with either leukaemia virus or lymphoma cells and subsequently reject challenge transplants of lymphoma cells, but viral immunisation still allows the possibility of viral infection of host cells of such a nature as to provoke host cell production of a specific antigen, which is the effective immunising agent.

The chemical nature and localisation in the cells of tumour specific antigens is not known but at least for the Moloney lymphoma antigen there is evidence that much of the antigen is on or near the cell surface (HAUGHTON, personal communication). In biological terms, these antigens are similar in behaviour to weak histocompatibility antigens. Various methods may be used to demonstrate their presence either *in vitro,* using complement fixation, fluorescein labelled antibody binding, and cytotoxic tests or *in vivo* by the induction of immune responses as measured by resistance to viral-induced tumour formation or to challenge with tumour transplants.

Where viral and host cell antigens can be studied separately, as with the polyoma virus, it has been found that it is only the immune response mounted by the body against the host cell-produced antigen which will result in rejection of tumour cells. The anti-viral immune response is not effective in protecting the host against challenge with tumour cells.

The immune resistance to tumour cells induced by these antigens is mediated by a cellular response, similar in general nature to that employed by the body in rejecting foreign tissue grafts. Humoral antibodies apparently do not play a singificant role in tumour cell rejection except possibly in the case of rejection of leukaemic cells.

It is apparent that during the development of a tumour one of three possibilities may occur (DEFENDI and ROOSA, 1964). 1. The emerging tumour cells may lack any distinguishing foreign antigens or the body may be unable to recognise and respond to such antigens and in this situation the proliferation of the tumour cells will continue unchecked by any host immune reaction. 2. If only weak foreign antigens occur in the tumour cells or if the host response to antigens is weak, some resistance to tumour proliferation may occur, which may exhibit itself in the form of a reduced growth rate of the tumour or in a prolongation of the latent period to tumour development. 3. If tumour antigens are strong and if host recognition and response systems are active, the first emerging tumour cells may have their growth completely inhibited or the tumour cells may be destroyed, in which case no tumours will develop.

From what has been said in this introduction it should be possible to cause an increased incidence of some tumours, or a shortening of the latent period to tumour development in animals by applying various procedures which will diminish host immune responses, particularly cellular immune responses. In this regard it is of considerable interest that many carcinogenic agents exert toxic effects on lymphoid cells and depress immune responses (MALMGREN, BENNISON and MCKINLEY, 1952; LINDER, 1962; and PREHN, 1963). It has been suggested that this depression of immune responses by chemical carcinogens may not be merely a side effect of these carcinogens but an essential part of the mechanism by which some chemical carcinogens operate. It may be essential in all carcinogenic situations involving the emergence of potentially antigenic tumour cells, that host immune responses be depressed at the critical time when the first cells are being converted to neoplastic cells. These questions have been discussed recently by PREHN (1963).

It seems difficult to imagine that any agent, whether immune response or cytotoxic drug, could be 100% effective in destroying tumour cells. Indeed it is well known that very few established tumours can be eliminated by measures designed to kill cells, e.g. irradiation or chemical agents, no matter how effective these may be. As will be recounted shortly, the evidence suggests, rather surprisingly, that immune responses *are* effective in preventing tumour formation. Why do not a few percent of resistant cells always succeed in breaking through these immune defences, and by proliferation, form a tumour? The explanation probably lies in the fundamental difference between the situation existing in an animal carrying an established tumour and the situation in an animal in which the first few tumour cells are emerging and attempting to proliferate. For reasons not understood at present it seems that during tumour development, before progressive tumour growth can be guaranteed, a critical size limit in the tumour cell population must be attained. To take a theoretical example, it may be that a tumour population needs to attain a size of 1000 cells before survival and progressive proliferation of this population is assured. If for some reason only 100 cells can be developed, this population may be unable to proliferate further and may remain dormant at this size or may ultimately die. It is difficult to envisage what mechanisms might determine such a situation, but the density of tumour cell population in one focus might be relevant for this might allow many important cell to cell interactions to occur. Such tumour cell crowding might be of critical importance in establishing a microenvironment containing optimal levels of metabolites for the growth of developing tumour cells, or might produce local concentrations of toxic products resulting in a growth advantage of the tumour cells over surrounding normal cells.

Under some circumstances, it has been shown that the transplantation of a single neoplastic cell to a normal animal will result in progressive tumour cell growth, ultimately killing the animal. However it is much more usual to find that there is a critical number (quite large) of tumour cells which must be transplanted to a recipient if a transplanted tumour is to result. Transplantation of fewer tumour cells than this critical number will not produce tumours and may in fact immunise the animal against further tumour cell challenge. Even mixing an adequate number of tumour cells with a population of normal cells may result in failure of the tumour cells to transplant—again raising the question of critical tumour cell population density, or crowding, as a factor allowing initial tumour growth.

Whatever the reasons responsible, it is now well established that the mere fact that some tumour cells are present in an animal does not mean that tumour formation is inevitable. It is at this initial stage in development of a tumour that an immune response by the host against the first few tumour cells may be able to prevent tumour development.

As has been shown, the thymus influences immune responses particularly those involving cellular responses of the tissue rejection, or hypersensitivity type. It should be possible then to demonstrate that the thymus influences tumour formation in those instances where the emerging tumour cells are antigenic. Many experiments have now shown that the thymus does affect this type of carcinogenesis.

The polyoma virus elicits in the host animal not only antibodies against viral antigen (anti-haemagglutinins) but also cellular immune responses against the viral induced host cell antigen. As was stated earlier, the immune response of animals to polyoma induced tumours is mediated by a cellular response to the polyoma virus induced host cell antigen, and not by the circulating anti viral antibodies. DEFENDI and KOPROWSKI (1959) working with the newborn hamster demonstrated that the induction of tumours by polyoma virus was delayed and the incidence of tumours reduced if these animals were previously injected with lymphocytes from adult hamsters immunised against polyoma virus. DEFENDI, ROOSA and KOPROWSKI (1964) in subsequent work showed that thymectomy at birth, followed a week later by injection of polyoma virus, led to a higher incidence of liver haemangiomata and death, than in control virus-infected hamsters. In the thymectomised hamsters with tumours, there was also a higher incidence of multiple tumours of different organs—liver, heart, kidney and at the injection site—than in sham operated hamsters with tumours. However in the group of thymectomised hamsters injected with polyoma virus it was possible to show that the level of circulating antibody to polyoma virus was as high as in sham operated virus-infected animals.

VANDEPUTTE et al. (1963) reported that neonatal thymectomy of rats rendered them more susceptible to tumour induction by the polyoma virus. When thymectomy or sham operation was performed at birth and the rats infected with polyoma virus 2—3 weeks later, 25% of the thymectomised rats but none of the sham operated rats developed tumours.

A similar type of result has been obtained by MILLER, TING and LAW (1964) and TING and LAW (1965) in polyoma induced tumour formation in mice. It was shown in C57Bl mice that while neonatal thymectomy depressed antibody formation against polyoma virus itself, thymectomy at three days of age did not affect the development of anti-viral antibody (TING and LAW, 1965). However in C57Bl mice, thymectomy at three days of age with subsequent injection of polyoma virus four days later, resulted in 90% of the thymectomised mice developing parotid gland tumours (mean latent period 69 days) versus only 6% in the sham operated virus infected mice (mean latent period to tumour development 118 days). This difference in tumour incidence was not related to any general decline in the health of the thymectomised mice, as body weight increase was normal in the mice thymectomised at three days of age. However, lymphocyte levels were lower in the thymectomised mice than in sham operated mice in the pretumour development period (MILLER, TING and LAW, 1964).

A second technique can be used to demonstrate immunological deficiencies in thymectomised mice in relation to their response to polyoma virus. Prior injection of polyoma virus elicits immunological responses to both viral and host cell antigens. When such mice are later challenged by transplants of polyoma-induced tumour cells, many of these mice fail to develop transplanted tumours, due to rejection of the transplanted cells (HABEL, 1961; SACKS, 1961). However mice thymectomised at birth, then injected with polyoma virus, and later challenged with polyoma cells all developed transplanted tumours, indicating their failure to develop a normal immune response to the tumour cell antigen (TING and LAW, 1965). Thymectomy at four weeks of age did not prevent virus-injected mice from developing a normal cellular immune response when challenged with tumour cells. When three days old (C57Bl $\times$ C3H)F_1 mice were thymectomised then grafted with whole C57Bl thymus grafts and virus injected one month later, they exhibited a normal capacity to reject challenge polyoma tumour cell transplants. This did not occur when virus injection was made only one week after thymus grafting.

In a recent study, LAW and TING (1965) demonstrated that polyoma virus achieved the same titres when injected into control C57Bl mice as in C57Bl mice thymectomised at three days of age. However the incidence of polyoma-induced tumours was again strikingly higher in the thymectomised mice than in the control groups. The excess incidence of tumours in the thymectomised mice was prevented by the injection of adult syngeneic spleen cells or by grafting C57Bl thymus tissue or C57Bl thymus tissue in millipore diffusion chambers.

This has provided clear evidence that the normal resistance of the host is against the cellular antigen of the polyoma system and further that this immune resistance is dependent on a thymic humoral factor in order to be effective.

In a recent study, KIRSCHSTEIN, RABSON and PETERS (1964) reported that human adenovirus 12 was unable to produce tumours in normal BALB/c and C3H/HeN mice. However in neonatally thymectomised mice of these strains, 8 of 48 mice developed subcutaneous tumours at the site of injection of the virus.

This latter finding is of considerable interest and suggests that neonatal thymectomy may be a very useful ancillary technique for use in investigating the potential carcinogenic properties of other human and animal viruses when it is necessary to use a test animal which is of a different species from that of the source of the virus.

As described earlier, many tumours induced by chemical carcinogens are antigenic in the isologous or autochthonous animal. MILLER, GRANT and ROE (1963) investigated the effect of thymectomy at three days of age on mice, which subsequently were painted at five weeks of age with 50 μgm of benzopyrene twice weekly for twenty weeks. By 160 days after the application of benzopyrene, papillomata had developed in approximately 50% of the thymectomised mice but in only 5% of sham thymectomised mice. In the thymectomised mice fewer papillomata regressed and more tended to become malignant than in control mice. The tumours also grew more rapidly in the thymectomised mice and reached a larger size than in the control mice.

Similarly MAISIN (1964) reported that multiple thymus grafts in L strain mice inhibited the development of skin cancers following painting with 20 methylcholanthrene. This author also reported that a similar inhibitory effect on carcinogenesis resulted when homogenates of neonatal L strain thymus where injected into carcinogen-treated mice.

GRANT and MILLER (1965) have also reported that 20 methylcholanthrene, when injected into C57Bl mice thymectomised at 3 days of age produced sarcomata more rapidly than in sham operated mice, although the final incidence of tumours was identical in both types of animal. The growth rate of established sarcomata in both types of animal appeared to be identical. No histological differences were observed between the sarcomata arising in the two types of host.

DEFENDI and ROOSA (1964) reported a study on C3H/Bi mice which were thymectomised at seven days of age and then given 350 r whole body irradiation at three weeks of age. At the age of six to seven months groups of these mice were injected with either methylcholanthrene or 3, 4—9, 10 dibenzanthracene. In the methylcholanthrene injected mice, fibrosarcomata appeared earlier and in a higher percentage of the thymectomised mice than in the control mice given methylcholanthrene alone. A similar but less marked trend was observed in the dibenzanthracene treated thymectomised and irradiated mice. Tumours in the thymectomised mice were larger than in control mice but once the tumours were established, the actual growth rates of the tumours appeared to be similar in the two types of animal. It was also observed in sections of the tumours that the fibrosarcomata in control mice were surrounded by a rim of lymphoid and plasma cells. No cellular infiltration was observed around the periphery of tumours arising in thymectomised animals.

Since chemical carcinogens themselves tend to depress immune responses, it is possible that the administration of chemical carcinogens combined with adult thymectomy might produce a degree of depression of immune responses severe enough to have a significant effect on carcinogenesis. Recently, NISHIZUKA, NAKAKUKI and USUI (1965) have reported such a study in which neonatal Swiss mice were injected with 20 methylcholanthrene and then thymectomised when aged 35—55 days. In male mice subjected to this combined treatment, 17 of 28 mice developed liver tumours whereas only 5 of 21 male mice treated with the carcinogen alone developed liver tumours. The incidence of lung, mammary and reticular tumours in these mice was not affected by thymectomy.

From these experiments it is clear that immune responses of the host can be important in determining whether or not tumours develop in response to either chemical or viral initiating agents. It also seems clear in situations where the emerging tumour cells are antigenic, that thymectomy, by reducing the host's immune competence, increases the frequency and shortens the latent period of tumour development, whilst thymus grafting restores normal host immune responses and a normal susceptibility to tumour development.

What importance do these facts have for the development of the typical case of cancer in man or animals? We know very little about the antigenic content of the average *spontaneous* cancer cell in man or animals but unless the experimentally-induced tumours are very misleading, it seems likelv that some at least of the spontaneous cancers of man and animals will be found to have similar foreign antigens. If so, then the host immune responses should be of considerable importance in determining the emergence or suppression of such cancer cells. Certain features of the natural history of cancer in man suggest the operation of tumour inhibiting influences. For example, preneoplastic lesions and *carcinomata in situ* are recognisable in many tissues and some of these are known to have a very long latent period before conversion to frank neoplasia. Similarly, the outgrowth of metastases may be delayed for many years after the removal of a primary tumour. Such behaviour of tumour cells "cannot be explained in terms of their known rates of proliferation for if even one" tumour cell was present and able to proliferate unchecked, it can be calculated that this one cell could form a large tumour mass within weeks or at most months. Obviously there are mechanisms in the body which are capable of holding tumour cell proliferation in check for long periods and some of these may well be immune mechanisms.

One of the characteristics of cancer in man is that the frequency of most types of cancer rises logarithmically with age (or more exactly with the log of the age) (ARMITAGE and DOLL, 1954). In general, a similar situation exists in animals—the older the animal the more likelihood of cancer development. Many factors in the ageing animal might allow the more ready emergence and proliferation of cancer cells but in the context of the present discussion we shall confine our attention to the nature of immune processes in the ageing animal.

Until recently little systematic study has been made on the immune reactivity of the aged animal. However in the case of the mouse there are now indications that, at least in some strains, ageing is associated with a distinct fall in immune competence. As referred to earlier, we have made a preliminary survey of immune responses in various mouse strains using the response to a single antigen, sheep red cells, as the index of immune competence. This particular antigen was chosen since it has been shown that agglutinin formation to sheep red cells is one of the immune responses sensitive to thymectomy. In C57Bl mice it was found that antibody titres in response to primary injection of sheep red cells were very low in early life but rose to a maximum in early adult life (2—3 months of age). However by 12 months of age (middle age) a distinct fall in titres was observed and by 18 months (old age) the agglutinin response was markedly lower than in early adult life (Fig. 32). This diminution in responsiveness was slightly more marked in the initial (19S) response than in the later (7S) response. A similar but less pronounced decline in agglutinin responses with advancing age was noted also in (AKR $\times$ C57Bl)F_1 mice. By contrast, no fall in agglutinin responses to sheep red cells was noted, even in advanced old age, in C3H mice. These data suggest that in some strains immune responses at least to some antigens, markedly decline with age. Possibly if other antigens were employed a decline in responsiveness might be observed in other strains currently appearing not to show a decline in immune responsiveness with age.

Is the degree of reduction in immune responsiveness just described for old C57Bl mice, severe enough to be of significance in permitting the proliferation of antigenic tumour cells which would normally be suppressed? This question has been examined by TELLER et al. (1964) who showed that old Swiss mice also exhibited some depression in immune responses and reticulo-endothelial activity. They challenged young and old Swiss mice with human tumour transplants and found that some old Swiss mice permitted the proliferation of these transplanted tumour cells whereas the young Swiss mice uniformly rejected the transplanted cells, probably by immunological recognition of, and reaction to, the foreign (histocompatibility) antigens of the tumour cells. More studies of this type are needed before a complete picture can be obtained of the reactivity of old mice to the transplantation of foreign tumour cells but the data obtained so far suggest that if antigenic tumour cells were to occur in an old animal, the animal might have great difficulty in eliminating them, using immune rejection mechanisms.

What are the reasons for the decline in immune responsiveness in old mice? This question has been analysed by MAKINODAN and PETERSON (1964) who found a similar fall with age in the agglutinin response of mice to sheep red cells to that just described in C57Bl mice. They demonstrated that the spleens of these old mice contained fewer cells capable of being stimulated to proliferate and produce antibody by the injected sheep red cells. Confirmation of this age reduction in the number of cells capable of reacting with sheep red cells has been obtained by MILLER (1965 a) and DIENER (personal communication) who showed, using the Jerne plaque system for demonstrating 19S producing cells, that fewer plaque forming cells were present in the spleens of old animals than in younger animals.

As described earlier, it seems doubtful whether the decline in immune competence in old age is due primarily to failing thymus function. Certainly, grafting of old animals with multiple neonatal thymus grafts led to no improvement in the immune response to sheep red cells. It seems more likely that the primary cause is a failing production of antigenically competent cells and/or a decline in the efficiency of the antigen trapping and processing reticulo-endothelial cells. However a decreased thymic output of cells or a decrease in thymic humoral factor production in old age may contribute to this end result.

Granted that declining thymus function may not play a major role in determining depressed immune responses in old age, thymectomy in earlier life undoubtedly accentuates the severity of these other age changes. It seems reasonable to expect therefore that thymectomy should be followed by an increased incidence of various spontaneous tumours in old age. No systematic study seems to have been made of the effect of thymectomy in early life on the *spontaneous* incidence of various tumours in old age, but such a study is urgently needed.

It was noted by earlier workers who investigated the role of the thymus in lymphoid leukaemia development, that although thymectomy prevented lymphoid leukaemia development, the thymectomised mice did develop late in life a significant incidence of myeloid leukaemia and reticulum cell sarcomata, and other unusual tumours were described (FURTH, 1946; GROSS, 1960; NAKAKUKI and NISHIZUKA, 1964; KUNII and FURTH, 1964). These findings are difficult to interpret in high leukaemia strain mice because thymectomy prolongs the life span of these mice beyond that normally seen. In recent experiments on mice of the high leukaemia strain

(AKR × C3H)F_1 we observed that all sham operated mice had died from lymphoid leukaemia by the age of 18 months. In thymectomised (AKR × C3H)F_1 mice it was observed that early death from lymphoid leukaemia was completely prevented and although 15% of these mice ultimately did develop lymphoid leukaemia, it occurred later in life (METCALF, WIADROWSKI and BRADLEY, 1965). As a consequence, the thymectomised mice lived an average of 6 months longer than did the sham operated mice. It was observed that 50% of the thymectomised mice developed either myeloid leukaemia or reticulum cell sarcoma—diseases rarely seen in sham operated mice of this strain. The problem is why did these thymectomised mice develop these other reticular tumours? Would a normal (AKR × C3H)F_1 mouse, if it could live to two years of age, also be subject to the development of these tumours or does the normal mouse suppress the formation of myeloid leukaemia and reticulum cell sarcomata by immune mechanisms dependent on the thymus? The leukaemia viruses are known to be multi potent and they have been shown to induce lymphoid leukaemia in some strains but myeloid leukaemia and reticulum cell sarcoma in other strains (GROSS, 1963). It is likely that incipient myeloid leukaemia and reticulum cell sarcomata are present in some (AKR × C3H)F_1 mice but that these diseases are normally slow to develop and never have a chance to emerge as clinical diseases before the animals die with lymphoid leukaemia. However immune mechanisms may be operative in the normal (AKR × C3H)F_1 mouse suppressing the emergence of these neoplasms and a study is urgently needed of (AKR × C3H)F_1 mice which have been thymectomised in young adult life and then grafted with C3H thymus grafts. C3H thymus grafting has been reported not to restore susceptibility to lymphoid leukaemia development in thymectomised F_1 hybrid mice (LAW, 1959). These thymectomised F_1 hybrid mice grafted with C3H thymus grafts should live longer than unoperated (AKR × C3H)F_1 mice and if they do not die prematurely with lymphoid leukaemia, will they now develop myeloid leukaemia and reticulum cell sarcoma or will the grafted thymus by restoring immune competence prevent the emergence of these neoplasms?

Similar questions may be raised regarding the nature of the osteomata reported by MCENDY, BOON and FURTH (1944) to occur in old age in thymectomised mice of the high leukaemia strain AKR.

In the experiments described so far in this discussion, thymectomy has been found to lead to an increased incidence and/or a reduced latent period to tumour development. However two recent studies on the effect of thymectomy on carcinogenesis appear to be at variance with this conclusion.

PREHN (1964 a) found that thymectomy in adult life decreased the incidence of fibrosarcomata induced by the injection of methylcholanthrene. MARTINEZ (1964) reported that thymectomy at 6 days of age in female C3H/Bi mice reduced the incidence of mammary tumour development from 94.5% in control mice to 57.6%.

Both findings are difficult to interpret in view of the much larger volume of evidence relating thymectomy with an *increased* incidence of various tumours. It has been suggested that a reduction in tumour incidence following thymectomy might occur because the thymus normally produces substances with trophic properties for tumour cells.

This suggestion of a trophic effect of the thymus on tumour growth is the second of the two possible influences of the thymus on carcinogenesis mentioned at the beginning of this chapter. We have seen from the discussion of possible trophic functions of the thymus that the thymus may well release to the circulation lymphocyte breakdown products which might be of value for rapidly growing tissues e.g. cancer tissue.

Actually the concept of a trophic influence of the thymus dates back to the early days of thymus research when ROWNTREE et al. (1935) reported that extracts of thymus when injected repeatedly into rats caused profound growth increase. So far as we are aware this observation has never been confirmed and we certainly have never observed increased body growth in mice given repeated injections of thymus extract or carrying multiple thymus grafts.

SZENT-GYORGYI, HEGYELI and MCLAUGHLIN (1962) made a preliminary report suggesting that thymus tissue may contain both an inhibitory factor (retine) and a promoting factor (promine) with activity on the growth of transplanted tumour cells, but this report awaits confirmation.

There is at present so little positive experimental support for the concept that the thymus exerts a trophic influence on tumour cell growth that this concept must be regarded as purely speculative until confirmatory evidence is produced.

It is conceivable that the influence of thymectomy in reducing the incidence of breast tumours in C3H/Bi mice may involve questions of tolerance breakdown of a similar nature to those discussed for leukaemogenesis. C3H/Bi mice are infected neonatally with the Bittner virus and the data of MORTON (1964) and MORTON, GOLDMAN and WOOD (1965) suggest that they are in a tolerant immune state to the virus. It may be that breast tumours only emerge following breakdown in tolerance to the virus. If so, thymectomy, by delaying or preventing tolerance breakdown, might reduce the incidence of breast tumours. This concept is again purely speculative but may be worth keeping in mind with regard to the other vertically transmitted tumour viruses where questions of tolerance may arise.

Pursuing these concepts to their limit, it seems that there may be two distinct ways in which the thymus may influence carcinogenesis. 1. Where emerging tumour cells are antigenic, the thymus may mobilize an effective host immune response which either leads to suppression of these tumour cells or to a delay in cancer development. This situation may be present with certain carcinogenic viruses, e.g. polyoma virus, and with certain chemical carcinogens or certain dosage schedules of carcinogens. In these cases thymectomy will increase the incidence of cancer and shorten the latent period to cancer development. 2. Where tumour viruses are transmitted vertically e.g. the mammary tumour virus and the Gross virus, a tolerant state to the virus exists during which no carcinogenesis may be possible. Breakdown in tolerance occurs with the passage of time, after which time virus-host cell interaction, possibly combined with immune response damage, may lead to cancer cell formation. In this situation thymectomy may lead to a prolongation of the period of tolerance, and thus lead to a prolongation of the latent period to cancer development and a reduced incidence of cancer.

Summary

Many cancer cells (particularly those induced by chemical carcinogens and tumour viruses) contain antigens foreign to the host. Host immune responses to these foreign antigens are capable, under some circumstances, of preventing the emergence and growth of these cancer cells, thus delaying or preventing tumour development.

Thymectomy, by reducing host immune responses, has been shown to shorten the latent period to tumour development and to increase the incidence of tumours following exposure of animals to chemical carcinogens and tumour viruses.

In part at least, the thymic influence on host immune responses to antigenic cancer cells is mediated via a humoral factor.

Spontaneous cancer development in old age may also be related to declining thymus function and immune responses in old age, at least in those instances in which the cancer cells contain foreign antigens.

Chapter 10

General Discussion

The thymus is a compound organ comprised of lymphoid cells and a complex of epithelial and reticulum cells. The lymphoid cell population is renewed every few days by intense local lymphopoiesis which is regulated primarily by an intrinsic proliferative stimulus produced by the epithelial and reticulum cell complex. Fluctuation in the strength of this intrinsic proliferative stimulus determines the unique growth characteristics of the thymus. Strain and sex differences in thymus weight and mitotic activity are due, in part at least, to differences in the proliferative stimulus exerted by the epithelial reticulum cell complex. Thymic lymphopoiesis does not appear to be affected by antigenic stimulation.

Despite the intense lymphopoiesis in the thymus, the indications are that relatively few of the cells produced in the thymus ever leave the organ. It must be admitted that at present the purpose of the major portion of thymic lymphopoietic activity is unknown.

It has been suggested that the intense lymphopoietic activity in the organ may represent a mechanism used to generate, by random genetic variation at mitosis, lymphocytes with different immunological reactivity patterns, and that the accompanying intense thymic lymphocyte breakdown may represent the destruction of undesirable lymphocytes having reactivity patterns which would allow them to react with self antigens. The efficiency of this postulated thymic surveillance—destruction mechanism seems doubtful in view of the evidence from preleukaemic animals which shows that the thymus is in fact the site in which preleukaemic lymphoid cells survive much better than elsewhere in the body.

Alternatively it has been suggested that thymic lymphoid cells or lymphocyte breakdown products may have trophic functions in the general body economy either by regulating the proliferation and differentiation of other tissue cells or by providing building blocks for these cells. Although there is some evidence from isotopic reutilisation studies that lymphocyte breakdown material can be incorporated in other dividing cells, it is rather disconcerting for those holding this trophic concept of thymic lymphocyte function that neonatal thymectomy of germfree animals is *not* followed by observable changes in body growth or function. Similarly there is no experimental support for the suggestion that thymic lymphoid cells may serve as stem cells for other haemopoietic cell systems, e.g. for red cell or myeloid cell formation.

In spite of the present difficulty in proposing a satisfactory reason for most of the lymphopoiesis occurring in the thymus, it seems likely that some lymphoid cells do leave the organ and that these are a very valuable source of cells for the replacement of cells lost from the peripheral lymphoid organs and possibly for the introduction into these organs of cells with new immune reactivity potentials. The thymus probably serves therefore as a limited, but permanent, source of lymphoid cells which are of primary importance for the body in maintaining immune responses against foreign antigens, invading micro-organisms and developing antigenic tumour cells.

Of even greater importance is the non-cellular influence exerted by the thymus on the functional activity of the lymphoid cells in other lymphoid organs. This influence is in the form of a humoral factor which is probably elaborated by the epithelial and reticulum cells of the thymus. Its mode of action has not been completely established but it is likely to function by allowing or accentuating the response of competent lymphoid cells to antigenic stimulation by proliferation, producing clones of plasma cells secreting specific antibody to the antigen and clones of lymphoid cells, some at least of which are capable of eliciting cellular immune responses.

The question of whether there is but one thymic humoral factor (regulating thymic lymphopoiesis, lymphoid and plasma cell, antigen initiated, proliferation and influencing leukaemogenesis) or whether there are a multiplicity of thymic factors was discussed exhaustively at a recent conference (CIBA Conference on the Thymus, 1965). It was even suggested that the thymus may secrete humoral factors regulating myeloid cells and having other functions. In view of the multiple and diverse nature of secretions from the pituitary, adrenal and salivary glands and the electronmicroscopic evidence of heterogeneity in the thymic epithelial cells, the possibility should not be dismissed lightly that the thymus does indeed secrete more than one humoral factor. The cellular events in which a non cellular thymic factor has been implicated are shown schematically in Figure 44. Although future work may indicate the existence of multiple factors, at present it is still possible to hold to the simple concept that there is but one humoral factor and that the different phenomena influenced by the humoral factor reflect qualitative differences in the target cells responding to stimulation. For example, the necessity for antigen to be present in addition to thymic humoral factor before lymph node lymphoid cells proliferate whilst thymic lymphoid cells apparently do not need antigen priming, may indicate not the existence of two separate factors but merely the existence of fundamental differences in the nature of the two cell types involved. This situation with thymic humoral fac-

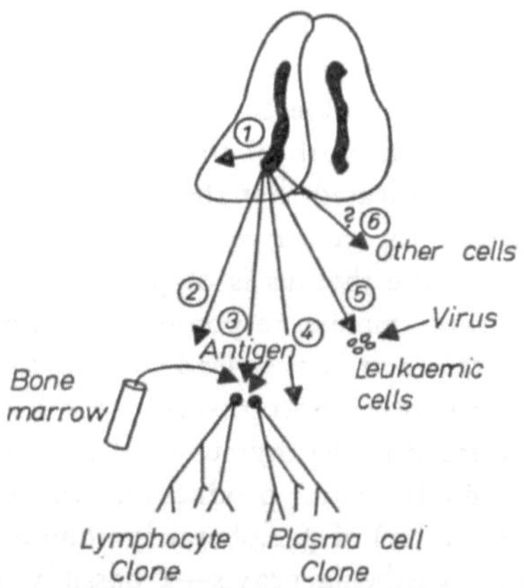

Fig. 44. Schematic diagram listing possible thymic humoral factors and their sites of action. Factors 1, 2, 3, 4 and 5 might be a single factor whose action produces a varying end result according to the nature of the target cell being stimulated. (1) Intrinsic proliferative stimulus. (2) Competence inducing factor. (3) Factor stimulating antigen initiated lymphopoiesis. (4) Factor stimulating antigen initiated plasma cell proliferation. (5) Lymphoid leukaemia inducing factor. (6) Action on other cells e. g. myelopoiesis inhibitory factor?

tor would then parallel the protean effects of cortisone on different cells in the body.

After removal of the thymus, particularly if thymectomy is performed early in life, severe immunological deficiencies develop, leading ultimately to premature death of the animal. In this sense the thymus is one of the vital organs of the body. However the thymus may not regulate *all* immune responses and it is possible that some types of immune response either may not need thymic stimulation or may be regulated by anologues of the thymus (e.g. the Bursa of Fabricius in chickens, the appendix and possibly the tonsils). Some have postulated that under some circumstances lymph nodes themselves may come to contain cells exerting a function similar to that of the thymic epithelial and reticulum cells. However there is no functional proof of this latter postulate which is based merely on superficial morphological resemblances between epithelial and reticular thymic cells and cells occasionally appearing in the lymph nodes.

The immune competence of the animal is of particular relevance to the question of carcinogenesis for it now appears that many cancer cells are antigenic for the host, and that the normal animal may protect itself against cancer development by identifying newly developed cancer cells as being foreign and by eliminating or suppressing them using immune mechanisms. It has been suggested by BURNET (1962) that this process of immune suppression of cancer cells may be the biological reason for the existence and development of the homograft rejection mechanism in mammals. Any factor tending to depress the body's immune defences would render the animal hypersusceptible to cancer development. Experimental studies in animals have confirmed the truth of these postulates, at least for viral and chemical carcinogens, and have indicated that the thymus is the foundation stone on which the body's immune system for cancer cell elimination rests.

If the thymus is of primary importance for the development and sustenance of normal immune responses against infections and cancer cells, does abnormal function of the thymus ever lead to autoimmune diseases in which the body's lymphoid tissues attack other host tissues? This situation might arise if self-reactive lymphoid cells emerged in the thymus itself (or were not eliminated there) or alternatively if thymic humoral factor production was excessive and allowed abnormal reactivity (self-reactivity) of peripheral lymphoid cells. It is true that thymectomy often cures cases of myasthenia gravis—a possibly autoimmune disease—and that in this disease the thymus has abnormal foci of immunologically reactive cells within the organ itself. However the beneficial effects of thymectomy in myasthenia gravis or other autoimmune diseases does not necessarily prove that these diseases were *initiated* by the thymus, for thymectomy may merely cause a general dampening down of all immune responses (including autoimmune responses), thus improving the clinical condition of the patient in a manner similar to that achieved by cortisone therapy. Further development of the concept of thymic initiation of autoimmune disease must await definite experimental proof of the existence of such a postulated sequence of events.

At least in rodents, the thymus occupies a central role in the development of lymphoid leukaemia. This role is quite the reverse of the previous functions discussed since it is the presence of the thymus rather than the removal of the organ which is responsible for disease development. Although much is understood of the aetiology and development of lymphoid leukaemia in rodents, the part played by the thymus is still incompletely understood Lymphoid leukaemia probably is usually intitiated by infection by one of the family of lymphoid leukaemia-inducing viruses. The affected lymphoid cells have been shown to pass through stages of dependency, responsiveness and autonomy to the thymic influence. Although the initial changes in this sequence may not need to occur in cells actually within the thymus, the first cells to reach the fully autonomous leukaemic state do so in the thymus. This suggests the operation of special short range influences within the thymus permitting or determining neoplasia development in these lymphoid cells and there is no direct proof that any humoral factor is involved in leukaemogenesis. However elevated levels of a lymphocytosis stimulating factor (probably thymic in origin) have been demonstrated in preleukaemic and leukaemic mice and humans and some leukaemogenesis experiments suggest the operation of a humoral factor. Whether the intrinsic thymic lymphopoietic stimulus is involved in leukaemogenesis is even less certain. The peculiar susceptibility of thymic lymphoid cells to neoplastic change may result from the presence of high titres of virus in the thymus, the rapid rate of division or special nature of thymic lymphoid cells, or because infection of the epithelial and reticulum cell elements of the thymus may be an essential part of the disease process. Whatever the mechanisms involved in the thymic influence on leukaemogenesis, the prevention of lymphoid leukaemia development in mice by thymectomy is one of the most dramatic and readily repeatable experiments it is possible to perform in the field of carcinogenesis.

Does the thymus in the neonatal animal perform any special or unique functions not performed in adult life? This suggestion has been raised repeatedly, and it has been claimed that the lymphopenia and depressed immune responses following neonatal thymectomy indicate some special function of the thymus at this time. This has led to the suggestion that the thymus may only export cells in the neonatal period or that only neonatal lymphoid cells need a thymic humoral factor.

We are firmly of the opinion that there is no significant difference between the function of the thymus in neonatal and adult life. As has been shown, adult thymectomy leads to exactly the same type of lymphocyte depletion and immune deficiencies as does neonatal thymectomy, the difference being merely one of the speed of development and the severity of these changes. The rapidity and severity of changes following neonatal thymectomy appear to be related to the lymphocyte depleted state of the newborn animal and its immunological immaturity (or inexperience) rather than to any difference in thymus function at this age. In adult animals if a similar degree of lymphopenia is produced by irradiation, thymectomy has an equally rapid and equally profound effect on the immune responses. In this context it is of particular significance that the length of time thymic humoral factor needs to be present to confer immune reactivity on lymphoid cells is strikingly similar in the newborn animal and the adult thymectomised animal. Thus thymectomy at 3 days of age has little immediate effect on immune responses, implying that three day's exposure to thymic humoral factor (from day 0 to day 3 of life) allows the lymphoid cells to function normally in the *immediate* post thymectomy period. In adult irradiated and thymectomised mice, thymus grafts similarly need only to be present for a few days to restore immune competence (at least temporarily). These similar time relationships strongly suggest that exactly the same cellular processes are operative in the neonatal and adult animal and that both are equally dependent on, and responsive to, a thymic influence. This still leaves open the possibility of a greater cell export from the thymus in neonatal life than in adult life.

It is now appreciated that the thymus, far from being a vestigial or functionless organ, is intimately involved in the body's defence systems against infection and cancer and that the thymus plays an important role in lymphoid leukaemia development. This knowledge is new and the field of thymus research is being expanded rapidly. We should not close our minds to the possibility that even now we do not know all there is to be learned of the functions of the thymus. It may be that the thymus has many other functions in the body quite unrelated to the lymphoid system and we must be prepared to design experiments to investigate this possibility.

References

AISENBERG, A. C., B. WILKES, and B. H. WAKSMAN: The production of runt disease in rats thymectomised at birth. J. exp. Med. **116**, 759 (1962).

ANDREASEN, E., and S. CRISTENSEN: Rate of mitotic activity in lymphoid organs of rat. Anat. Rec. **103**, 401 (1949).

ARCHER, O., and J. C. PIERCE: Role of thymus in development of the immune response. Fed. Proc. **20**, 26 (1961).

— —, B. W. PAPERMASTER, and R. A. GOOD: Reduced antibody response in thymectomised rabbits. Nature **195**, 191 (1962).

ARGYRIS, B. F.: Loss of acquired tolerance to skin homografts in mice. Transplant. Bull. **30**, 140 (1962).

— Effect of thymus grafts, spleen cell injection and sublethal irradiation on homograft tolerance in mice. Transplantation **3**, 350 (1965).

ARMITAGE, P., and R. DOLL: The age distribution of cancer and a multistage theory of carcinogenesis. Brit. J. Cancer **8**, 1 (1954).

ARNASON, B. G., C. DE VAUX ST. CYR, and P. GRABAR: Immunoglobulin abnormalities of the thymectomised rat. Nature (Lond.) **199**, 1199 (1963).

—, B. D. JANKOVIC, B. H. WAKSMAN, and C. WENNERSTEIN: Role of the thymus in immune reactions in rats. II Suppressive effect of thymectomy at birth on reactions of delayed (cellular) hypersensitivity and the circulating small lymphocyte. J. exp. Med. **116**, 177 (1962).

ARNESEN, K.: The secretory apparatus in the thymus of mice. Acta pathol. microbiol. scand. **43**, 339 (1958).

— Preleukemic and early leukemic changes in the thymus of mice. Acta pathol. microbiol. scand. **43**, 350 (1958 a).

AUERBACH, R.: Experimental analysis of the origin of cell types in the development of the mouse thymus. Develop. Biol. **3**, 336 (1961).

— Thymus: its role in lymphoid recovery after irradiation. Science **139**, 1061 (1963).

— Developmental studies of mouse thymus and spleen. N.C.I. Monogr. **11**, 23 (1963 a).

AXELRAD, A. A.: Antigenic behaviour of lymphoma cell populations in mice as revealed by the spleen colony method. Progress in Experimental Tumour Res. **6**, (1965).

—, and H. C. VAN DER GAAG: Susceptibility to lymphoma induction by Gross' passage A virus in C3Hf/Bi mice of different ages: Relation to thymic cell multiplication and differentiation. J. Nat. Canc. Inst. **28**, 1065 (1962).

AZAR, H. A.: Bacterial infection and wasting in neonatally thymectomised rats. Proc. Soc. exper. Biol. Med. **116**, 817 (1964).

BARCLAY, T. J., I. L. WEISSMAN, and H. S. KAPLAN: Discussion session in "The Thymus". Eds. V. Defendi and D. Metcalf. Philadelphia: Wistar Institute Press 1964.

BARNES, D. W. H., C. E. FORD, P. L. T. ILBERY, K. W. JONES, and J. F. LOUTIT: Murine leukaemia. Acta Union int. Cancr. **15**, 544 (1959).

BIELSCHOWSKY, M., B. J. HELYER, and J. B. HOWIE: Spontaneous haemolytic anaemia in mice of the NZB/BL strain. Proc. Univ. Otago Med. School. **37**, 9 (1957).

BIERRING, F.: Quantitative investigations on the lymphomyeloid system in thymectomised rats. In CIBA Symposium "Haemopoiesis. Cell production and its regulation". Eds. G. E. W. Wolstenholme and M. O'Connor. London: Churchill 1960.

— The lymphocyte content of the bone marrow in thymectomised-lymphadenectomised rats. Acta anat. 55, 9 (1963).

BILLINGHAM, R. E., and W. K. SILVERS: Some biological differences between thymocytes and lymphoid cells. In "The Thymus". Eds. V. Defendi and D. Metcalf. Philadelphia: Wistar Institute Press 1964.

BJORNEBOE, M., H. GORMSEN, and F. LUNDQUIST: Further experimental studies on the role of plasma cells as antibody producers. J. Immunol. 55, 121 (1947).

BOYD, E.: Weight of thymus gland in health and in disease. Amer. J. Dis. Child. 43, 1162 (1932).

BRYANT, B. J.: Reutilisation of lymphocyte DNA by cells of intestinal crypts and regenerating liver. J. Cell Biol. 18, 515 (1963).

BURNET, M.: Role of the thymus and related organs in immunity. Brit. med. J. 2, 807 (1962).

BURNET, F. M., and M. C. HOLMES: Thymic changes in the mouse strain NZB in relation to the auto-immune state. J. Path. Bact. 88, 229 (1964).

— — Genetic investigations of autoimmune disease in mice. Nature 207, 368 (1965).

CAMBLIN, J. G., and J. B. BRIDGES: Effects of cell free extracts of thymus in leucopenic rats. Transplantation 2, 785 (1964).

CARNES, W. H., and H. S. KAPLAN: Relation of lymphoma induction to cortical differentiation in thymic grafts in irradiated C57Bl mice. Fed. Proc. 15, 510 (1956).

CLAMAN, H. N., and W. McDONALD: Thymus and x-radiation in the termination of acquired immunological tolerance in the adult mouse. Nature 202, 712 (1964).

—, and D. W. TALMAGE: Thymectomy: prolongation of immunological tolerance in the adult mouse. Science 141, 1193 (1963).

CLARK, S. L.: The thymus in mice of strain 129/J studied with the electron microscope. Amer. J. Anat. 112, 1 (1963).

— The penetration of proteins and colloidal materials into the thymus from the blood stream. In "The Thymus". Eds. V. Defendi and D. Metcalf. Philadelphia: Wistar Institute Press 1964.

— Cytological evidences of secretion in the thymus. In CIBA Symposium "The Thymus: Experimental and Clinical Studies". Eds. R. Porter and G. E. W. Wolstenholme. London: J. & A. Churchill 1965. (In press)

COMSA, J.: Influence of purified thymus extracts on haemopoietic organs of guinea pigs irradiated with x-rays. C. R. Soc. Biol. 150, 516 (1956).

CRADDOCK, C. G., G. S. NAKAI, H. FUKUTA, and L. M. VANSLAGER: Proliferative activity of the lymphatic tissue of rats as studied with tritium-labeled thymidine. J. exp. Med. 120, 389 (1964).

—, T. RYTOMAA, and G. S. NAKAI: The transfer of labeled DNA from blood cells to regenerating liver. In "The Thymus in Immunobiology" Eds. R. A. Good and A. E. Gabrielsen. New York: Harper and Row 1964.

CROSS, A. M., E. LEUCHARS, and J. F. A. P. MILLER: Studies on the recovery of the immune response in irradiated mice thymectomised in adult life. J. exp. Med. 119, 837 (1964).

CUDKOWICZ, G., A. C. UPTON, L. H. SMITH, D. G. GOSSLEE, and W. L. HUGHES: An approach to the characterisation of stem cells in mouse bone marrow. Ann. N. Y. Acad. Sci. 114, 571 (1964).

DALMASSO, A. P., C. MARTINEZ, and R. A. GOOD: Studies of immunologic characteristics of lymphoid cells from thymectomised mice. In "The Thymus in Immunobiology". Eds. R. A. Good and A. E. Gabrielsen. Harper and Row, New York: 1964.

— —, K. SJODIN, and R. A. GOOD: Studies on the role of the thymus in immunobiology. Reconstitution of immunologic capacity in mice thymectomised at birth. J. exp. Med. 118, 1089 (1963).

DALTON, A. J., L. W. LAW, J. B. MOLONEY, and R. A. MANAKER: An electron microscope study of a series of murine lymphoid leukemias. J. Nat. Cancer Instit. 27, 747 (1961).

DAMESHEK, W.: Immunocytes and immunoproliferative disorders. In CIBA Symposium "The Thymus. Experimental and Clinical Studies." Eds. R. Porter and G. E. W. Wolstenholme. London: Churchill 1965.

DAY, E. D.: The immunochemistry of cancer. Springfield: Thomas 1965.

DEFENDI, V.: Effect of SV40 virus immunisation on growth of transplantable SV40 and polyoma virus tumors in hamsters. Proc. Soc. exper. Biol. Med. 113, 12 (1963).

—, and H. KOPROWSKI: Influence of adult lymphoid tissues on polyoma induced tumours. Nature 184, 1579 (1959).

—, and R. A. ROOSA: The role of the thymus in carcinogenesis. In "The Thymus". Philadelphia: Wistar Institute Press. Eds. V. Defendi and D. Metcalf 1964.

— —, and H. KOPROWSKI: Effect of thymectomy at birth on response to tissue, cells and virus antigens. In The Thymus in Immunobiology. Eds. R. A. Good and A. E. Gabrielsen. New York: Harper and Row 1964.

DE HARVEN, E.: Virus particles in the thymus of conventional and germfree mice. J. exp. Med. 120, 857 (1964).

DENT, P. B., R. D. A. PETERSON, and R. A. GOOD: A defect in cellular immunity during the incubation period of passage A leukemia in C3H mice. Proc. Soc. exp. Biol. Med. 119, 869 (1965).

DE SOMER, P., P. DENYS, and R. LEYTEN: Activity of a noncellular calf thymus extract in normal and thymectomised mice. Life Sciences 1, 810 (1963).

DIXON, F. J., W. O. WEIGLE, and J. C. ROBERTS: Comparison of antibody responses associated with the transfer of rabbit lymph node, peritoneal exudate and thymus cells. J. Immunol. 78, 56 (1957).

DOUGHERTY, T. F.: Effect of hormones on lymphatic tissue. Physiol. Rev. 32, 379 (1952).

—, M. L. BERLINER, G. L. SCHNEEBELI, and D. L. BERLINER: Hormonal control of lymphatic structure and function. Ann. N. Y. Acad. Sci. 113, 825 (1964).

DUPLAN, J. F., G. V. FOSCHI, and L. A. MANSON: The lymphocytosis stimulating factor (L.S.F.). Proc. Soc. exp. Biol. Med. 110, 426 (1962).

EAST, J., and D. M. V. PARROTT: Prevention of wasting in mice thymectomised at birth and their subsequent rejection of allogeneic leukemic cells. J. nat. Cancer Inst. 33, 673 (1964).

— —, F. C. CHESTERMAN, and A. POMERANCE: The appearance of a hepatotrophic virus in mice thymectomised at birth. J. exp. Med. 118, 1069 (1963).

— —, and J. SEAMER: The ability of mice thymectomised at birth to survive infection with lymphocytic choriomeningitis virus. Virology 22, 160 (1964).

FACHET, J., E. STARK, M. PALKOVITS, and K. VALLENT: Der Einfluß der Thymektomie auf die Lieberregeneration nach partieller Hepatektomie. Z. Zellforsch 60, 609 (1963).

FEFER, A., and G. J. V. NOSSAL: Abolition of neonatally-induced homograft tolerance in mice by sublethal irradiation. Transplant. Bull. 29, 445 (1962).

FICHTELIUS, K. E.: On the destination of thymus lymphocytes. In CIBA Symposium "Haemopoiesis. Cell Production and its Regulation". Eds. G. E. W. Wolstenholme and M. O'Connor. London: Churchill 1960.

—, and H. DIDERHOLM: Autoradiographic analysis of the accumulation of lymphocytes in wounds. Acta. pathol. microbiol. scand. 52, 11 (1961).

—, G. LAURELL, and L. PHILIPSSON: The influence of thymectomy on antibody formation. Acta. pathol. microbiol. scand. 51, 81 (1961).

FISHER, E. R.: Pathology of the thymus and its relation to human disease. In "The Thymus in Immunobiology" Eds. R. A. Good and A. E. Gabrielsen. New York: Harper and Row 1964.

FLIEDNER, T. M., M. KESSE, E. P. CRONKITE, and J. S. ROBERTSON: Cell proliferation in germinal centres of the rat spleen. Ann. N. Y. Acad. Sci. 113, 578 (1964).

FOLEY, E. J.: Antigenic properties of methylcholanthrene-induced tumors in mice of the strain of origin. Cancer Res. 13, 835 (1953).

FORD, C. E., and H. S. MICKLEM: The thymus and lymph nodes in radiation chimaeras Lancet 359 (1963).

FRIEDMAN, H.: Absence of antibody plaque forming cells in spleens of thymectomised mice immunised with sheep erythrocytes. Proc. Soc. exp. Biol. Med. 118, 1176 (1965).

FURTH, J.: Prolongation of life with prevention of leukemia by thymectomy in mice. J. Gerontol 1, 46 (1946).
— Parallel observations on the role of thymus in lymphopoiesis, immunocompetence and viral leukemogenesis. In CIBA Symposium "The Thymus. Experimental and Clinical Studies." Eds. R. Porter and G. E. W. Wolstenholme. London: Churchill 1965.
—, and M. C. BOON: The time and site of origin of the leukemic cell. A.A.A.S. Research Conference on Cancer 1944. Washington A.A.A.S. p. 129 (1945).
—, and M. C. KAHN: The transmission of leukemia of mice with a single cell. Amer. J. Cancer 31, 276 (1937).
GARDNER, W. U., T. F. DOUGHERTY, and W. L. WILLIAMS: Lymphoid tumors in mice receiving steroid hormones. Cancer Res. 4, 73 (1944).
GLANZMANN, E., and P. RINIKER: Essentielle Lymphocytophthise. Ein neues Krankheitsbild aus der Säuglingspathologie. Ann. paediat. 17, 1 (1950).
GLICK, B.: Extracts from the bursa of Fabricius—a lympho-epithelial gland of the chicken—stimulate the production of antibodies in bursectomised chickens. Poultry Science 39, 1097 (1960).
—, T. S. CHANG, and R. G. JAAP: The bursa of Fabricius and antibody production. Poultry Science 35, 224 (1956).
GLOBERSON, A., and M. FELDMAN: Role of the thymus in restoration of immune reactivity and lymphoid regeneration in irradiated mice. Transplantation 2, 212 (1964).
— — Antigenic specificity of benzo(a)pyrene induced sarcomas. J. nat. Cancer Inst. 32, 1229 (1964 a).
GOOD, R. A.: Agammaglolulinemia—A provocative experiment of nature. Bull. Univ. Minn. Hosp. Minn. Med. Found. 26, 1 (1954).
—, A. P. DALMASSO, C. MARTINEZ, O. K. ARCHER, J. C. PIERCE, and B. W. PAPERMASTER: The role of the thymus in development of immunologic capacity in rabbits and mice. J. exp. Med. 116, 773 (1962).
—, C. MARTINEZ, and A. E. GABRIELSEN: Clinical considerations of the thymus in immunobiology. In "The Thymus in Immunobiology". Eds. R. A. Good and A. E. Gabrielsen. New York: Harper and Row 1964.
GORDON, H. A.: Morphological and physiological characterisation of germfree life. Ann. N. Y. Acad. Sci. 78, 208 (1959).
GOWANS, J. L., and E. J. KNIGHT: The route of recirculation of lymphocytes in the rat. Proc. roy. Soc. B. 159, 257 (1964).
GRAFFI, A.: Experiments on the hematological diversity of viral mouse leukemias. In "Murine Leukemia". Monograph. National Cancer Institute. Bethesda 1965. (In press)
GRANT, G. A., and J. F. A. P. MILLER: Effect of neonatal thymectomy on the induction of sarcomata in C57Bl mice. Nature (Lond.) 205, 1124 (1965).
GREEN, I.: The regeneration of F_1 host cell spleen and thymus at ectopic sites in F_1 animals induced by implantation of parental spleen and thymus. J. exp. Med. 119, 581 (1964).
—, and K. BLOCH: Uptake of particulate matter within the thymus of adult and newborn mice. Nature (Lond.) 200, 1099 (1963).
GREGOIRE, C., and C. DUCHATEAU: A study on lympho-epithelial symbiosis in thymus; reactions of the lymphatic tissue to extracts and to implants of epithelial components of thymus. Arch. Biol. (Liege) 67, 269 (1956).
GROSS, L.: Pathogenic properties and "vertical" transmission of the mouse leukemia agent. Proc. Soc. exp. Biol. Med. 78, 342 (1951).
— Serial cell-free passage of a radiation-activated mouse leukemia agent. Proc. Soc. exp. Biol. Med. 100, 102 (1959).
— Effect of thymectomy on development of leukemia in C3H mice inoculated with leukemic "Passage" virus. Proc. Soc. exp. Biol. Med. 100, 325 (1959 a).
— Development of myeloid (chloro-)leukemia in thymectomised C3H mice following inoculation of lymphatic leukemia virus. Proc. Soc. exp. Biol. Med. 103, 509 (1960).
— Pathogenic potency and host range of the mouse leukemia virus. Acta haematol. 29, 1 (1963).
— Attempt at classification of mouse leukemia viruses. Acta haematol. 32, 81 (1964).

GRUTER, V. B., A. L. TRAPP, and V. L. SANGER: A lymphocytosis stimulating substance in Mongoloid plasma. Nature **207**, 306 (1965).

GYLLENSTEN, L.: Influence of thymus and thyroid on the postnatal growth of the lymphatic tissue in guinea pigs. Acta anat. Suppl. **18**, 17 (1953).

— Influence of thyroxin on regeneration of the lymphatic tissue after corticosteroid-induced involution. Acta pathol. microbiol. scand. **56**, 29 (1962).

HABEL, K.: Resistance of polyoma virus immune animals to transplanted polyoma tumors. Proc. Soc. exp. Biol. Med. **106**, 722 (1961).

— Polyoma tumor antigen in cells transformed in vitro by polyoma virus. Virology **18**, 553 (1962).

—, and B. E. EDDY: Specificity of resistance to tumor challenge of polyoma and SV_{40} virus-immune hamsters. Proc. Soc. exp. Biol. Med. **113**, 1 (1963).

HAMMAR, J. A.: The new views as to the morphology of the thymus gland and their bearing on the problem of the function of the thymus. Endocrinology **5**, 543 (1921).

HANNA, M. G.: An autoradiographic study of the germinal center in spleen white pulp during early intervals of the immune response. Lab. Investigation **13**, 95 (1964).

HARAN-GHERA, N., and H. S. KAPLAN: Lymphoma development in intrarenal thymus implants in thymectomised irradiated mice. Proc. Amer. Assoc. Cancer Res. **5**, 25 (1964).

HARRIS, J. E., D. W. BARNES, C. E. FORD, and E. P. EVANS: Cellular traffic of the thymus: Experiments with chromosome markers. Evidence from parabiosis for an afferent stream of cells. Nature (Lond.) **201**, 884 (1964).

—, and C. E. FORD: Cellular traffic of the thymus: Experiments with chromosome markers. Evidence that the thymus plays an instructional part. Nature (Lond.) **201**, 884 (1964).

HARRIS, T. M., J. RHOADS, and J. STOKES: A study of the role of the thymus and spleen in the formation of antibodies in the rabbit. J. Immunol. **58**, 27 (1948).

HELLSTROM, K. E., and G. MOLLER: Immunological and immunogenetic aspects of tumor transplantation. Progr. Allergy **9**, 158 (1965).

HOHN, E. O.: Action of certain hormones on the thymus of the domestic hen. J. Endocrinol. **19**, 282 (1959).

HOLMES, M. C., and M. BURNET: Thymic changes in NZB mice and hybrids. In CIBA Symposium "The Thymus. Experimental and clinical studies." Eds. R. Porter and G. E. W. Wolstenholme. London: Churchill 1965. (In press)

HOSHINO, T.: Electron microscopic studies of the epithelial reticular cells of the mouse thymus. Z. Zellforsch. **59**, 513 (1963).

HOTCHIN, J.: The biology of lymphocytic choriomeningitis infection: Virus-induced immune disease. Cold Spr. Harb. Symp. quant. Biol. **27**, 479 (1962).

HOWIE, J. B.: The influence of neonatal thymectomy and thymus grafting on spontaneous autoimmune disease in mice. In CIBA Symposium. "The Thymus. Experimental and Clinical Studies." Eds. R. Porter and G. E. W. Wolstenholme. London: Churchill 1965.

—, and B. J. HELYER: Autoimmune disease in mice. Ann. N. Y. Acad. Sci. **124**, 167 (1965).

HUMBLE, J. G., W. H. W. JAYNE, and R. J. V. PULVERTAFT: Biological interaction between lymphocytes and other cells. Brit. J. Haematol. **2**, 283 (1956).

HUMPHREY, J. H., D. M. V. PARROTT, and J. EAST: Studies on globulin and antibody production in mice thymectomised at birth. Immunology **7**, 419 (1964).

ILBERY, P. L. T., P. A. MOORE, S. M. WINN, and C. E. FORD: Chromosomes in murine preleukaemia. In "Cellular Basis and Aetiology of late Somatic Effects of Ionizing Radiation". New York: Academic Press 1962.

ISAKOVIC, K., S. B. SMITH, and B. H. WAKSMAN: Immunologic tolerance in thymectomised irradiated rats grafted with thymus from tolerant donors. Science **148**, 1333 (1965).

ISHIDATE, M., and D. METCALF: The pattern of lymphopoiesis in the mouse thymus after cortisone administration or adrenalectomy. Aust. J. exp. Biol. med. Sci. **41**, 637 (1963).

ITO, T., and T. HOSHINO: Studies on the influences of pregnancy and lactation on the thymus in the mouse. Z. Zellforsch. **57**, 667 (1962).

— — Influences of the gonad on the thymus in the mouse. Z. Anat. Entwickl. Gesch. **123**, 490 (1963).

ITO, Y., and F. B. WEINSTEIN: A factor in the serum of irradiated rats stimulating lymphoid tissue mitosis. J. nat. Cancer Inst. **29**, 229 (1962).

JANKOVIC, B. D., and S. LESKOWITZ: Restoration of antibody producing capacity in bursectomised chickens by bursal grafts in millipore chambers. Proc. Soc. exp. Biol. Med. **118**, 1164 (1965).

—, B. H. WAKSMAN, and B. G. ARNASON: Role of the thymus in immune reactions in rats I. The immunologic response to bovine serum albumin (antibody formation, Arthus reactivity and delayed hypersensitivity) in rats thymectomised or splenectomised at various times after birth. J. exp. Med. **116**, 159 (1962).

JERNE, K., A. A. NORDIN, and C. HENRY: The agar-plate technique for recognising antibody producing cells. In "Cell-Bound Antibodies". Eds. B. Amos and H. Koprowski. Philadelphia: Wistar Institute Press 1963.

JONEJA, M. G., and H. F. STICH: The survival of abnormal cells in the thymus of mice. Exp. Cell Res. **31**, 220 (1963).

JOSKE, R. A.: The effects of thymectomy on the lymphocyte count in patients with myasthenia gravis. Med. J. Australia **2**, 859 (1958).

KAPLAN, H. S.: Observations on radiation-induced lymphoid tumors of mice. Cancer Res. **7**, 141 (1947).

— Influence of thymectomy, splenectomy and gonadectomy on incidence of radiation-induced lymphoid tumors in strain C57Bl mice. J. nat. Cancer Inst. **11**, 83 (1950).

— On the etiology and pathogenesis of the leukemias: A review. Cancer Res. **14**, 535 (1954).

— The role of cell differentiation as a determinant of susceptibility to virus carcinogenesis. Cancer Res. **21**, 981 (1961).

— Interaction of occult leukaemogenic viruses with ionizing radiation and other external leukaemogenic agents in the induction of thymic lymphosarcoma in the mouse. In "The Thymus. Experimental and Clinical Studies". Eds. G. E. W. Wolstenholme and R. Porter. London: Churchill 1965.

—, M. B. BROWN, and J. PAULL: Influence of post irradiation thymectomy and of thymic implants on lymphoid tumor incidence in C57Bl mice. Cancer Res. **13**, 677 (1953).

— — — Influence of bone marrow injections on involution and neoplasia of mouse thymus after systemic irradiation. J. nat. Cancer Inst. **14**, 303 (1953 a).

—, B. B. HIRSCH, and M. B. BROWN: Genetic evidence of the origin of the tumor cells from the thymic grafts. Cancer Res. **16**, 434 (1956).

—, C. S. NAGAREDA, and M. B. BROWN: Endocrine factors and radiation-induced lymphoid tumors of mice. In Recent Progress in Hormone Research **10**, 293 (1954). Ed. G. Pincus. New York: Academic Press.

KINDRED, J. F.: Aquantitative study of the lymphoid organs of albino rats. Amer. J. Anat. **62**, 453 (1938).

KIRSCHSTEIN, R. L., A. S. RABSON, and E. A. PETERS: Oncogenic activity of adenovirus 12 in thymectomised BALB/c and C3H/HeN mice. Proc. Soc. exp. Biol. Med. **117**, 198 (1964).

KLEIN, G., H. O. SJOGREN, and E. KLEIN: Demonstration of host resistance against isotransplantation of lymphomas induced by the Gross agent. Cancer Res. **22**, 955 (1962).

— — —, and K. E. HELLSTROM: Demonstration of resistance against methylcholanthrene-induced sarcomas in the primary autochthonous host. Cancer Res. **20**, 1561 (1960).

KLEIN, J. J., A. L. GOLDSTEIN, and A. WHITE: Enhancement of in vivo incorporation of labeled precursors into DNA and total protein of mouse lymph nodes after administration of thymic extracts. Proc. nat. Acad. Sci. **53**, 812 (1965).

KOCH, M. A., and A. B. SABIN: Specificity of virus-induced resistance to transplantation of polyoma and SV_{40} tumors in adult hamsters. Proc. Soc. exp. Biol. Med. **113**, 4 (1963).

KUNII, A., and J. FURTH: Inhibition of lymphoma induction in virus-infected rats by thymectomy. An affinity of the lymphoma virus for myeloid cells. Cancer Res. **24**, 493 (1964).

LATARJET, R.: Carcinogenesis by leukaemic cell-free extracts in mice. In CIBA Symposium "Carcinogenesis. Mechanisms of Action". Eds. G. E. W. Wolstenholme and M. O'Connor. London: Churchill 1959.

LAW, L. W.: The effect of gonadectomy and adrenalectomy on the appearance and incidence of spontaneous lymphoid leukemia in mice. J. nat. Cancer Inst. **8**, 157 (1947).

LAW, L. W.: Increase in incidence of leukaemia in hybrid mice bearing thymic transplants from a high leukaemic strain. J. nat. Cancer Inst. 12, 789 (1952).
— Maternal influence in experimental leukemia in mice. Ann. N. Y. Acad. Sci. 57, 575 (1954).
— Some aspects of the etiology of leukemia. In Canadian Cancer Conference 3. Ed. R. W. Begg. New York: Academic Press 1959.
— Influence of foster-nursing in virus-induced and spontaneous leukemia in mice. Proc. Soc. exp. Biol. Med. 111, 615 (1962).
—, T. R. BRADLEY, and S. ROSE: Reversal of the thymus-dependent influence in radiation leukemogenesis of C57Bl mice. J. nat. Cancer Inst. 31, 1461 (1963).
—, T. B. DUNN, N. TRAININ, and R. H. LEVEY: Studies of thymic function. In "The Thymus". Eds. V. Defendi and D. Metcalf. Philadelphia: Wistar Institute Press 1964 a.
—, and J. H. MILLER: Observations on the effect of thymectomy on spontaneous leukemias in mice of the high leukemia strains RIL and C58. J. nat. Cancer Inst. 11, 253 (1950).
— — The influence of thymectomy on the incidence of carcinogen-induced leukemia in strain DBA mice. J. nat. Cancer Inst. 11, 425 (1950 a).
—, and M. POTTER: The behaviour in transplant of lymphocytic neoplasms arising from parental thymic grafts in irradiated, thymectomised hybrid mice. Proc. nat. Acad. Sci. 42, 160 (1956).
—, and R. C. TING: Immunologic competence and induction of neoplasms by polyoma virus. Proc. Soc. exp. Biol. Med. 119, 823 (1965).
—, N. TRAININ, R. H. LEVEY, and W. F. BARTH: Humoral thymic factor in mice: Further evidence. Science 143, 1049 (1964).
LEBLOND, C. P.: Classification of cell populations on the basis of their proliferative behaviour. National Cancer Institute Monograph No. 14. "Control of Cell Division and the Induction of Cancer", 119 (1964).
LEBLOND, C. P., and G. SAINTE-MARIE: Models for lymphocyte and plasmocyte formation. In CIBA Symposium "Haemopoiesis. Cell Production and its Regulation". Eds. G. E. W. Wolstenholme and M. O'Connor. London: Churchill 1960.
LEUCHARS, E., A. M. CROSS, and A. J. DAVIES: A cellular component of thymic function. Nature (Lond.) 203, 1189 (1964).
LEVEY, R. H., N. TRAININ, and L. W. LAW: Evidence for function of thymus tissue in diffusion chambers implanted in neonatally thymectomised mice. J. nat. Cancer Inst. 31, 199 (1963).
LEVINTHAL, J. D., and R. F. BUFFETT: Thymectomy and thymus grafts in mouse viral leukemia. Proc. Soc. exp. Biol. Med. 106, 426 (1961).
— —, and J. FURTH: Prevention of viral lymphoid leukemia of mice by thymectomy. Proc. Soc. exp. Biol. Med. 100, 610 (1959).
LIEBERMAN, M., and H. S. KAPLAN: Leukemogenic activity of filtrates from radiation-induced lymphoid tumors of mice. Science 130, 387 (1959).
LINDER, O. E.: Survival of skin homografts in methylcholanthrene-treated mice and in mice with spontaneous mammary cancers. Cancer Res. 22, 380 (1962).
LITTLE, J. R., G. BRECHER, T. R. BRADLEY, and S. ROSE: Determination of lymphocyte turnover by continuous infusion of H_3 thymidine. Blood 19, 236 (1962).
LOEWENTHAL, L. A., and C. SMITH: Studies on the thymus of the mammal. IV. Lipid-laden foamy cells in the involuting thymus of the mouse. Anat. Rec. 112, 1 (1952).
LORENZ, E., L. W. LAW, and C. C. CONGDON: The role of bone marrow and spleen in induced and spontaneous lymphatic leukaemia. In CIBA Symposium "Leukaemia Research". Ed. G. E. W. Wolstenholme. London: Churchill 1954.
LOUTIT, J. F.: Immunological and trophic functions of lymphocytes. Lancet 1106 (1962).
MACKAY, I. R., M. MASEL, and F. M. BURNET: Thymic abnormality in systemic lupus erythematosus. Aust. Ann. Med. 13, 5 (1964).
MACLEAN, L. D., S. J. ZAK, R. L. VARCO, and R. A. GOOD: Thymic tumor and acquired agammaglobulinemia—A clinical and experimental study of the immune response. Surgery 40, 1010 (1956).
MAISIN, J. H. F.: Role of thymus and thymus factors in the induction of 20 methylcholanthrene skin cancer in mice. Nature (Lond.) 202, 202 (1964).

MAKINODAN, T., and W. J. PETERSON: Growth and senescence of the primary antibody-forming potential of the spleen. J. Immunol. **93**, 886 (1964).
MALMGREN, R. A., B. E. BENNISON, and T. W. MCKINLEY Jr.: Reduced antibody titres in mice treated with carcinogenic and cancer chemotherapeutic agents. Proc. Soc. exp. Biol. Med. **79**, 484 (1952).
MARCHESI, V. T., and J. L. GOWANS: The migration of lymphocytes through the endothelium of venules in lymph nodes: an electron microscope study. Proc. roy. Soc. (B) **159**, 283 (1964).
MARSHALL, A. H. E., and R. G. WHITE: The immunological reactivity of the thymus. Brit. J. exp. Path. **42**, 379 (1961).
MARTINEZ, C.: Effect of early thymectomy on development of mammary tumors in mice. Nature (Lond.) **203**, 1188 (1964).
—, A. P. DALMASSO, M. BLAESE, and R. A. GOOD: Runt disease produced in thymectomised F_1 mice injected with parental strain lymphoid cells. Proc. Soc. exp. Biol. Med. **111**, 404 (1962).
—, J. KERSEY, B. W. PAPERMASTER, and R. A. GOOD: Skin homograft survival in thymectomised mice. Proc. Soc. exp. Biol. Med. **109**, 193 (1962 a).
MATSUYAMA, M., M. WIADROWSKI, and D. METCALF: Autoradiographic analysis of lymphopoiesis and lymphocyte migration in mice bearing multiple thymus grafts. J. exp. Med. **123**, 559 (1966).
MCENDY, D. P., M. C. BOON, and J. FURTH: On the role of the thymus, spleen and gonads in the development of leukemia in a high leukemia stock of mice. Cancer Res. **4**, 377 (1944).
MCINTIRE, K. R., S. SELL, and J. F. A. P. MILLER: Pathogenesis of the post-neonatal thymectomy wasting syndrome. Nature **204**, 151 (1964).
METCALF, D.: A lymphocytosis stimulating factor in the plasma of chronic lymphatic leukaemic patients. Brit. J. Cancer **10**, 169 (1956).
— Further studies on the plasma lymphocytosis stimulating factor in chronic lymphatic leukaemia and some other disease states. Brit. J. Cancer **10**, 431 (1956 a).
— The thymic origin of the plasma lymphocytosis stimulating factor. Brit. J. Cancer **10**, 442 (1956 b).
— Long-term effects of whole body irradiation on lymphocyte homeostasis in the mouse. Rad. Research **10**, 313 (1959).
— The thymic lymphocytosis stimulating factor and its relation to lymphatic leukemia. In Third Canadian Cancer Conference. Ed. R. W. Begg. New York: Academic Press 1959 a.
— The effect of thymectomy on the lymphoid tissues of the mouse. Brit. J. Haematol. **6**, 324 (1960).
— Adrenal cortical function in high—and low—leukemia strains of mice. Cancer Res. **20**, 1347 (1960 a).
— Leukaemogenesis in AKR mice. In CIBA Symposium. "Tumour Viruses of Murine Origin". Eds. G. E. W. Wolstenholme and M. O'Connor. London: Churchill 1962.
— A thymus responsive phase in leukaemogenesis in AKR mice. Nature (Lond.) **195**, 88 (1962 a).
— The autonomous behaviour of normal thymus grafts. Aust. J. exp. Biol. med. Sci. **41**, 437 (1963).
— The fate of parental preleukemic cells in leukemia-susceptible and leukemia-resistant F_1 hybrid mice. Cancer Res. **23**, 1774 (1963 a).
— Spleen graft growth in splenectomised mice. Aust. J. exp. Biol. med. Sci. **41**, 51 (1963 b).
— The thymus and lymphopoiesis. In "The Thymus in Immunobiology". Eds. R. A. Good and A. E. Gabrielsen. New York: Harper and Row 1964.
— Functional interactions between the thymus and other organs. In "The Thymus". Eds. V. Defendi and D. Metcalf. Philadelphia: Wistar Institute Press 1964 a.
— Thymus grafts and leukemogenesis. Cancer Res. **24**, 1952 (1964 b).
— Effect of pregnancy and testosterone on thymus grafts. Transplantation **2**, 541 (1964 c).
— Restricted growth capacity of multiple spleen grafts. Transplantation **2**, 387 (1964 d).

Metcalf, D.: The nature and regulation of lymphopoiesis in the normal and neoplastic thymus. In CIBA Symposium "The Thymus: Experimental and Clinical Studies". Eds. R. Porter and G. E. W. Wolstenholme. London: Churchill 1965 (in press).
— Multiple thymus grafts in aged mice. Nature 208, 87 (1965 a).
— Delayed effect of thymectomy in adult life on immunological competence. Nature (Lond.) 208, 1336 (1965 b).
—, and R. Bradley: The growth and erythropoietic activity of spleen grafts placed under the kidney capsule. Aust. J. exp. Biol. med. Sci. 43, 229 (1965).
—, and M. Ishidate: Periodic Acid-Schiff positive giant cells in the mouse thymus cortex. Nature (Lond.) 191, 305 (1961).
— — PAS-positive reticulum cells in the thymus cortex of high and low leukaemia strains of mice. Aust. J. exp. Biol. med. Sci. 40, 57 (1962).
—, and K. Nakamura: Lymphocyte production and differentiation in the preleukaemic mouse thymus. In "The Morphological Precursors of Cancer". Ed. L. Severi. Perugia: Perugia University Press 1962.
— —, and M. Wiadrowski: Patterns of cellular differentiation in spontaneous and transplanted lymphomata in mice. Aust. J. exp. Biol. med. Sci. 43, 413 (1965).
—, N. Sparrow, K. Nakamura, and M. Ishidate: The behaviour of thymus grafts in high and low leukaemia strains of mice. Aust. J. exp. Biol. med. Sci. 39, 441 (1961).
—, and R. Wakonig-Vaartaja: Stem cell replacement in normal thymus grafts. Proc. Soc. exp. Biol. Med. 115, 731 (1964).
— — Host cell repopulation of normal spleen grafts. Lancet 1012 (1964 a).
— —, and T. R. Bradley: The growth and repopulation of thymus grafts placed under the kidney capsule. Aust. J. exp. Biol. med. Sci. 43, 17 (1965).
—, and M. Wiadrowski: Autoradiographic analysis of lymphocyte proliferation in the thymus and in thymic lymphoma tissue. Cancer Res. 26, 483 (1966).
— —, and R. Bradley: Analysis of the role of the thymus in leukemia development using thymectomy and thymus grafts. In "Murine Leukemia". Monograph National Cancer Institute (in press) (1965).
Miller, J. F. A. P.: Role of the thymus in murine leukaemia. Nature 183, 1069 (1959).
— Studies on mouse leukaemia. The role of the thymus in leukaemogenesis by cell-free leukaemic filtrates. Brit. J. Cancer 14, 93 (1960).
— Studies on mouse leukaemia. The fate of thymus homografts in immunologically tolerant mice. Brit. J. Cancer 14, 244 (1960 a).
— Recovery of leukaemogenic agent from non-leukaemic tissues of thymectomised mice. Nature 187, 703 (1960 b).
— Immunological function of the thymus. Lancet 2, 748 (1961).
— Analysis of the thymus influence in leukaemogenesis. Nature 191, 248 (1961 a).
— Etiology and pathogenesis of mouse leukemia. Adv. Cancer Res. 6, 292 (1961 b).
— Effect of neonatal thymectomy on the immunological responsiveness of the mouse. Proc. roy. Soc. (B) 156, 415 (1962).
— Immunological significance of the thymus of the adult mouse. Nature (Lond.) 195, 1318 1962.
— Role of the thymus in transplantation immunity. Ann. N. Y. Acad. Sci. 99, 340 (1962 b).
— Role of the thymus in virus-induced leukaemia. In CIBA Symposium "Tumour Viruses of Murine Origin". Eds. G. E. W. Wolstenholme and M. O'Connor. London: Churchill 1962 c).
— The thymus and the development of immunologic responsiveness. Science 144, 1544 (1964).
— Effect of thymic ablation and replacement. In "The Thymus in Immunobiology". Eds. R. A. Good and A. E. Gabrielsen. New York: Harper and Row 1964 a.
— The thymus in relation to the development of immunological capacity. In CIBA Symposium "The Thymus. Experimental and Clinical Studies". Eds. R. Porter and G. E. W. Wolstenholme. London: Churchill 1965. (In press)
— Effect of thymectomy in adult mice on immunological responsiveness. Nature (Lond.) 208, 1337 (1965 a).

MILLER, J. F. A. P., M. BLOCK, D. T. ROWLANDS, and P. KIND: Effect of thymectomy on hemopoietic organs of the opossum "embryo". Proc. Soc. exp. Biol. Med. **118**, 916 (1965).

—, S. M. A. DOAK, and A. M. CROSS: Role of the thymus in recovery of the immune mechanism in the irradiated adult mouse. Proc. Soc. exp. Biol. Med. **112**, 785 (1963).

—, G. A. GRANT, and F. J. C. ROE: Effect of thymectomy on the induction of skin tumours by 3,4-benzopyrene. Nature (Lond.) **199**, 920 (1963).

—, and J. G. HOWARD: Some similarities between the neonatal thymectomy syndrome and graft-versus-host disease. J. Reticuloendothelial Soc. **1**, 369 (1964).

—, E. LEUCHARS, A. M. CROSS, and P. DUKOR: Immunologic role of the thymus in radiation chimeras. Ann. N. Y. Acad. Sci. **120**, 205 (1964).

—, R. C. TING, and L. W. LAW: Influence of thymectomy on tumor induction by polyoma virus in C57Bl mice. Proc. Soc. exp. Biol. Med. **116**, 323 (1964).

MITCHELL, J., W. MCDONALD, and G. J. V. NOSSAL: Autoradiographic studies on the immune response III Differential lymphopoiesis in various organs. Aust. J. exp. Biol. med. Sci. **41**, 411 (1963).

MOLLER, G.: 19S antibody production against soluble lipopolysaccharide antigens by individual lymphoid cells in vitro. Nature **207**, 1166 (1965).

MONEY, W. L., P. TYPOND, and R. W. RAWSON: The growth and function of thiouracil-induced thyroid tumors transplanted into non inbred rats thymectomised at birth. Cancer Res. **25**, 423 (1965).

MORTON, D. L.: Acquired immunological tolerance to spontaneous mammary adenocarcinomas following neonatal infection with mammary tumor agent. Proc. Amer. Assoc. Cancer Res. **5**, 46 (1964).

—, L. GOLDMAN, and D. A. WOOD: Immunological tolerance to spontaneous mammary adenocarcinomas. Proc. Amer. Assoc. Cancer Res. **6**, 47 (1965).

MOWBRAY, J. F.: Ability of large doses of an alpha-2 plasma protein fraction to inhibit antibody production. Immunology **6**, 217 (1963).

MUELLER, A. P., H. R. WOLFE, and R. K. MEYER: Precipitin production in chickens. XXI Antibody production in bursectomised chickens and in chickens injected with 19-nor-testosterone on the fifth day of incubation. J. Immunol. **85**, 172 (1960).

MURPHY, J. B.: The effect of castration, theelin and testosterone on the incidence of leukemia in a Rockefeller Institute strain of mice. Cancer Res. **4**, 622 (1944).

MURRAY, R. G., and P. A. WOODS: Studies on the fate of lymphocytes. The migration and metamorphosis of in situ labeled thymic lymphocytes. Anat. Rec. **150**, 113 (1964).

NAKAKUKI, K., and Y. NISHIZUKA: Induction of leukemia by x-ray irradiation, administration of estrogen and thymus transplantation in F_1 hybrid mice: A/Jax and AKR cross. Acta haematol. Jap. **25**, 786 (1962).

— — Age changes in the thymus in two high-leukaemia strains of mice, SL and AKR and in their F_1 hybrids. Nature (Lond.) **197**, 1217 (1963).

— — Effect of adult thymectomy on lymphoid tissues and the pathology of leukemia in mice of high-leukemia strains. Gann **55**, 509 (1964).

NAKAMOTO, A.: The influence of the thymus on blood, especially on lymphocytes. I Effects of thymectomy on the peripheral blood and lymph nodes. Acta haematol. Jap. **20**, 179 (1957).

— The influence of the thymus on blood, especially on lymphocytes. II Influence of thymus extracts on the peripheral blood lymphocytes. Acta haematol. Jap. **20**, 187 (1957 a).

NAKAMURA, K., and D. METCALF: Quantitative cytological studies on thymic lymphoid cells in normal, preleukaemic and leukaemic mice. Brit. J. Cancer **15**, 306 (1961).

NISHIZUKA, Y., K. NAKAKUKI, and M. USUI: Enhancing effect of thymectomy on hepatotumorigenesis in Swiss mice following neonatal injection of 20-methylcholanthrene. Nature **205**, 1236 (1965).

NOSSAL, G. J. V.: Studies on the rate of seeding of lymphocytes from the intact guinea pig thymus. Ann. N. Y. Acad. Sci. **120**, 171 (1964).

—, G. L. ADA, and C. M. AUSTIN: Antigens in immunity. IV. Cellular localisation of I^{125} and I^{131} labelled flagella in lymph nodes. Aust. J. exp. Biol. med. Sci. **42**, 311 (1964).

NOSSAL, G. J. V., and J. M. MITCHELL: The thymus in relation to immunological tolerance. In "The Thymus. Experimental and Clinical Studies". Eds. R. PORTER and G. E. W. WOLSTENHOLME. London: Churchill 1965 (in press).

OKANO, H., A. KUNII, and J. FURTH: An electron microscopic study of leukemia induced rats with Gross virus. Cancer Res. **23**, 1169 (1963).

OLD, L. J., E. A. BOYSE, D. A. CLARKE, and E. A. CARSWELL: Antigenic properties of chemically induced tumors. Ann. N. Y. Acad. Sci. **101**, 80 (1962).

— —, and E. STOCKERT: The G (Gross) leukemia antigen. Cancer Res. **25**, 813 (1965).

OSOBA, D., and J. F. A. P. MILLER: Evidence for a humoral thymus factor responsible for the maturation of immunological faculty. Nature **199**, 653 (1963).

— — The lymphoid tissue and immune responses of neonatally thymectomised mice bearing thymus tissue in millipore diffusion chambers. J. exp. Med. **119**, 177 (1964).

PATON, D. N., and A. GOODALL: Contribution to the physiology of the thymus. J. Physiol. **31**, 49 (1904).

PEPPER, F. J.: The effect of age, pregnancy and lactation on the thymus gland and lymph nodes of the mouse. Endocrin. **22**, 335 (1961).

— Transplantation of thymic tissue in inbred strains of mice. Endocrin. **22**, 349 (1961 a).

PETERSON, R. D. A., R. HENDRICKSON, and R. A. Good: Reduced antibody forming capacity during the incubation period of Passage A leukemia in C3H mice. Proc. Soc. exp. Biol. Med. **114**, 517 (1963).

PREHN, R. T.: Function of depressed immunologic reactivity during carcinogenesis. J. nat. Cancer Inst. **31**, 791 (1963).

— A clonal selection theory of chemical carcinogenesis. J. nat. Cancer Inst. **32**, 1 (1964).

— (personal communication) (1964 a).

—, and J. M. MAIN: Immunity to methylcholanthrene-induced sarcomas. J. nat. Cancer Inst. **18**, 769 (1957).

REBUCK, J. W., H. I. COFFMAN, G. B. BLUHM, and C. L. BARTH: A structural study of reticulum cell and monocyte production with quantitation of lymphocyte modulation of nonmultiplicative types to histiocytes. Ann. N. Y. Acad. Sci. **113**, 595 (1964).

REIF, A. E., and J. M. ALLEN: The AKR thymic antigen and its distribution in leukemias and nervous tissues. J. exp. Med. **120**, 413 (1964).

REIKE, W. O.: The *in vivo* reutilisation of lymphocytic and sarcoma DNA by cells growing in the peritoneal cavity. J. Cell Biol. **13**, 205 (1962).

REINHARDT, W. O., and J. M. YOFFEY: Thoracic duct lymph and lymphocytes in the guinea pig. Effects of hypoxia, fasting, evisceration and treatment with adrenaline. Amer. J. Physiol. **187**, 493 (1956).

ROWE, W. P., P. H. BLACK, and R. H. LEVEY: Protective effect of neonatal thymectomy on mouse LCM infection. Proc. Soc. exp. Biol. Med. **114**, 248 (1963).

ROWLEY, D. A., and F. W. FITCH: The mechanism of tolerance produced in rats to sheep erythrocytes. II The plaque-forming cell and antibody response to multiple injections of antigen begun at birth. J. exp. Med. **121**, 683 (1965).

ROWNTREE, L. G., J. H. CLARK, A. M. HANSON, and A. STEINBERG: Biologic effects of thymus extract (Hanson). Accruing acceleration in growth and development in five successive generations of rats under continuous treatment with thymus. Arch. int. Med. **56**, 1 (1935).

RUDALI, G., J. F. DUPLAN, and R. LATARJET: Latency of leukosis in Ak mice injected with leukemic acellular Ak extract. C. R. Acad. Sci. (Paris) **242**, 837 (1956).

SACHS, L.: Tumor transplantation in mice inoculated with polyoma virus. Exp. Cell. Res. **24**, 185 (1961).

SAINTE-MARIE, G.: Antigen penetration into the thymus. J. Immunol. **91**, 840 (1963).

SAXTON, J. A., M. C. BOON, and J. FURTH: Observations on the inhibition of development of spontaneous leukemia by underfeeding. Cancer Res. **4**, 401 (1944).

SCHOOLEY, J. C., and L. S. KELLY: Influence of the thymus on the output of thoracic duct lymphocytes. In "The Thymus in Immunobiology". Eds. R. A. Good and A. E. Gabrielsen. New York: Harper and Row 1964.

SHELTON, E., and A. J. DALTON: Electron microscopy of emperipolesis. J. Biophys. Biochem. Cytology **6**, 513 (1959).

SIEGLER, R., and M. A. RICH: Unilateral histogenesis of AKR thymic lymphoma. Cancer Res. **23**, 1669 (1963).

SJOGREN, H. O., I. HELLSTROM, and G. KLEIN: Transplantation of polyoma virus-induced tumors in mice. Cancer Res. **21**, 329 (1961).

SLETTENMARK, B., and E. KLEIN: Cytotoxic and neutralization tests with serum and lymph node cells of isologous mice with induced resistance against Gross lymphomas. Cancer Res. **22**, 947 (1962).

STICH H. F.: Mosaic composition of preneoplastic lesions and malignant neoplasms. Exp. Cell Res. Suppl. **9**, 277 (1963).

STONER, R. D., and W. M. HALE: Antibody production by thymus and Peyer's patches intraocular transplants. J. Immunol. **75**, 203 (1955).

STRAUSS, A. J. L.: Autoimmune concomitants of myasthenia gravis: studies of disease specificity and relevance to thymic pathology. In CIBA Symposium "The Thymus. Experimental and Clinical Studies". Eds. R. Porter and G. E. W. Wolstenholme. London: Churchill 1965. (In press)

—, B. C. SEEGAL, K. C. HSU, P. M. BURKHOLDER, W. L. NASTUK, and K. E. OSSERMAN: Immunofluorescent demonstration of a muscle binding, complement-fixing serum globulin fraction in myasthenia gravis. Proc. Soc. exp. Biol. Med. **105**, 184 (1960).

STUTMAN, O., and S. B. ZINGALE: Immunological reactivity of thymic autografts in rat. Proc. Soc. exp. Biol. Med. **117**, 389 (1964).

SZENBERG, A., and N. L. WARNER: Breakdown of polyvalent tolerance in the chicken by thymic grafts. Nature **198**, 1012 (1963).

SZENT-GYORGYI, A., A. HEGYELI, and J. A. McLAUGHLIN: Constituents of the thymus gland and their relation to growth, fertility and cancer. Proc. nat. Acad. Sci. **48**, 1439 (1962).

TAYLOR, R. B.: Decay of immunological responsiveness after thymectomy in adult life. Nature (Lond) **208**, 1334 (1965).

TELLER, M. N., G. STOHR, W. CURLETT, M. L. KUBISEK, and D. CURTIS: Aging and cancerigenesis I Immunity to tumor and skin grafts. J. nat. Cancer Inst. **33**, 649 (1964).

TELKKA, A., and H. TIER: Influence of thymus suspension on mitotic rate in the thymus, liver and outer orbital gland of the rat. Acta. pathol. microbiol. scand. **36**, 323 (1955).

THORBECKE, G. J., and M. W. COHEN: Immunological competence and responsiveness of the thymus. In "The Thymus". Eds. V. Defendi and D. Metcalf. Philadelphia: Wistar Institute Press 1964.

—, H. A. GORDON, B. S. WOSTMANN, M. WAGNER, and J. A. REYNIERS: Lymphoid tissue and serum gamma globulin in young germfree chickens. J. infect. Dis. **101**, 237 (1957).

—, and F. J. KEUNING: Antibody formation *in vitro* by hematopoietic organs after subcutaneous and intravenous immunisation. J. Immunol. **70**, 129 (1953).

TING, R. C., and L. W. LAW: The role of thymus in transplantation resistance induced by polyoma virus. J. nat. Cancer Inst. **34**, 521 (1965).

TOTH, B.: Development of malignant lymphomas by cell-free filtrates prepared from a chemically induced mouse lymphoma. Proc. Soc. exp. Biol. Med. **112**, 873 (1963).

TROWELL, O. A.: Radiosensitivity of the cortical and medullary lymphocytes in the thymus. Int. J. Rad. Biol. **4**, 163 (1961).

UPTON, A. C., and J. FURTH: The effects of cortisone on the development of spontaneous leukemia in mice and on its induction by irradiation. Blood **9**, 686 (1954).

VANDEPUTTE, M., P. DENYS, R. LEYTEN, and P. DE SOMER: The oncogenic activity of the polyoma virus in thymectomised rats. Life Sci. **1**, 475 (1963).

VOLKMAN, A., and J. L. GOWANS: The production of macrophages in the rat. Brit. J. exp. Path. **46**, 50 (1965).

— — The origin of macrophages from bone marrow in the rat. Brit. J. exp. Path. **46**, 62 (1965 a).

WAKSMAN, B. H., B. G. ARNASON, and B. D. JANKOVIC: Role of the thymus in immune reactions in rats. III Changes in the lymphoid organs of thymectomised rats. J. exp. Med. **116**, 187 (1962).

WARNER, N. L.: The immunological role of different lymphoid organs in the chicken. II The immunological competence of thymic cell suspensions. Aust. J. exp. Biol. med. Sci. **42**, 401 (1964).

WARNER, N. L., and A. SZENBERG: Immunologic studies on hormonally bursectomised and surgically thymectomised chickens: Dissociation of immunologic responsiveness. In "The Thymus in Immunbiology". Eds. R. A. GOOD and A. E. GABRIELSEN. New York: Harper and Row 1964.

WEISS, L.: Electron microscopic observations on the vascular barrier in the cortex of the thymus in the mouse. Anat. Rec. 145, 413 (1963).

WHANG, J., E. FREI, J. H. TJIO, P. P. CARBONE, and G. BRECHER: The distribution of Philadelphia chromosome in patients with chronic myeloid leukemia. Blood 22, 664 (1963).

WILSON, R., K. SJODIN, and M. BEALMAR: Thymus studies in germfree (Axenic) mice. In "The Thymus". Eds. V. Defendi and D. Metcalf. Philadelphia: Wistar Institute Press 1964.

WOOLLEY, G. W., and C. C. LITTLE: The incidence of adrenal cortical carcinoma in gonadectomised male mice of the extreme dilution strain. Cancer Res. 5, 211 (1945).

YOFFEY, J. M.: Cellular equilibria in blood and blood-forming tissues. In Homeostatic Mechanisms. Brookhaven Symp. Biol. 10, 1 (1957).

Monographs already published

SCHINDLER, R., Lausanne: Die tierische Zelle in Zellkultur (Volume 1).

Neuroblastomas — Biochemical Studies. Edited by C. BOHUON, Villejuif (Volume 2, Symposium).

HUEPER, W. C., Bethesda: Occupational and Environmental Cancers of the Respiratory System (Volume 3).

GOLDMAN, L., Cincinnati: Laser Cancer Research (Volume 4).

METCALF, D., Melbourne: The Thymus. Its Role in Immune Responses, Leukemia Development and Carcinogenesis (Volume 5).

Malignant Transformation by Viruses. Edited by W. H. KIRSTEN, Chicago (Volume 6, Symposium).

In production

MOERTEL, CH. G., Rochester: Multiple Primary Malignant Neoplasms: Their Incidence and Significance (Volume 7).

New Trends in the Treatment of Cancer. Edited by L. MANUILA, S. MOLES and P. RENTCHNICK, Geniva (Volume 8, Symposium).

LINDENMANN, J., Zürich / A. KLEIN, Gainesville, Florida: Immunological Aspects of Viral Oncolysis (Volume 9).

NELSON, R. S., Houston: Radioactive Phosphorus in the Diagnosis of Gastrointestinal Cancer (Volume 10).

FREEMANN, R. G., Houston/J. M. KNOX, Paris: Treatment of Skin Cancer (Volume 11).

In preparation

DENOIX, P., Villejuif: Le traitement des cancers du sein.

FISHER, E. R., Pittsburgh: Ultrastructure of Human Normal and Neoplastic Prostate.

FUCHS, W. A., Bern: Lymphography and Tumordiagnosis.

GRUNDMANN, E., Wuppertal-Elberfeld: Morphologie und Cytochemie der Carcinogenese.

HALPERN, B., Paris/PEJSACHOWICZ, Paris: L'agrégation des cellules cancéreuses in vitro.

HAYWARD, J. L., London: Cancer of the Breast: Hormonal Changes.

KERN, G., Köln: Carcinoma in situ.

MARTZ, G., Zürich: Hormonbehandlung der Tumoren.

MATHÉ, G., Villejuif: Les essais d'éradication des leucémies aiguës.

NEWMAN, M. K., Detroit: Neuropathies and Myopathies associated with Occult Malignancies.

PACK, G. T., New York: Clinical Aspects of Cancer Immunity and Cancer Susceptibility.

PACK, G. T., New York / A. H. ISLAMI, New York: Tumors of the Liver.

RITZMAN, S. E., Galveston / W. C. LEVIN, Galveston: The Syndrome of Macroglobulinemia.

STEWARD, J. K., Manchester: Tumors in Children.

WEIL, R., Lausanne: Biological and structural properties of polyoma virus and its DNA.

ZILBER, L. A., Moskva: Virogenetic Theory of Cancer Origin.

MIX
Papier aus verantwortungsvollen Quellen
Paper from responsible sources
FSC® C105338

If you have any concerns about our products,
you can contact us on
ProductSafety@springernature.com

In case Publisher is established outside the EU,
the EU authorized representative is:
Springer Nature Customer Service Center GmbH
Europaplatz 3, 69115 Heidelberg, Germany

Printed by Libri Plureos GmbH
in Hamburg, Germany